The Power of Connection

Relational-Cultural Theory (RCT) proposes that all people grow through and toward relationships throughout their lifespan. RCT challenges prevailing theories that depict the "separate self" as the hallmark of maturity. Rather than movement toward autonomy and separation, RCT suggests we develop ever more differentiated ways of connecting. An increase in growth-fostering relationships results in: a sense of vitality and zest; increasing clarity about ourselves and others; augmented creativity and ability to take action; an experience of worth and empowerment; and a desire for more connectedness with others. Disconnections are inevitable in relationships and RCT focuses on relational resilience, the ways people can re-establish positive and growth-fostering relationships.

RCT further emphasizes the importance of cultural and societal forces in causing either growth-fostering connection or destructive disconnection. This volume explores the process of change in therapy and in other relationships; how race and other forms of stratification create pain; and how people develop resilience and strength in relationships characterized by mutuality.

This book was based on a special issue of *Women and Therapy*.

Judith V. Jordan is Director of the Jean Baker Miller Training Institute and an Assistant Professor at the Harvard Medical School. She has written and lectured widely on topics of relational psychology, empathy, mutuality, the psychology of women, shame and the power of connection.

The Power of Connection

Recent Developments in
Relational-Cultural Theory

Edited by Judith V. Jordan

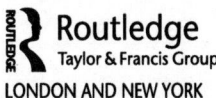
LONDON AND NEW YORK

First published 2010 by Routledge
2 Park Square, Milton Park, Abingdon, Oxon, OX14 4RN

Simultaneously published in the USA and Canada
by Routledge
270 Madison Avenue, New York, NY 10016

Routledge is an imprint of the Taylor & Francis Group, an informa business

© 2010 Taylor & Francis

Typeset in Times by Value Chain, India
Printed and bound in Great Britain by TJI Digital, Padstow, Cornwall

All rights reserved. No part of this book may be reprinted or reproduced or utilised in any form or by any electronic, mechanical, or other means, now known or hereafter invented, including photocopying and recording, or in any information storage or retrieval system, without permission in writing from the publishers.

British Library Cataloguing in Publication Data
A catalogue record for this book is available from the British Library

ISBN10: 0-415-56810-2
ISBN13: 978-0-415-56810-4

CONTENTS

INTRODUCTION

Recent Developments in Relational-Cultural Theory   1
Judith V. Jordan

SECTION ONE: RCT AND THERAPY

Introduction to Section One: RCT and Therapy   5

1. Creative Moments in Relational-Cultural Therapy   6
   Irene Pierce Stiver
   Wendy Rosen
   Janet Surrey
   Jean Baker Miller

2. What Changes in Therapy? Who Changes?   29
   Natalie S. Eldridge
   Janet L. Surrey
   Wendy P. Rosen
   Jean Baker Miller

3. Strengthening Resilience in a Risky World:
   It's All About Relationships   49
   Linda M. Hartling

4. When Racism Gets Personal: Toward Relational Healing   69
   Maureen Walker

5. How Therapy Helps When the Culture Hurts   84
   Maureen Walker

SECTION TWO: THE IMPORTANCE OF POWER

Introduction to Section Two: The Importance of Power   103

6. How Change Happens: Controlling Images, Mutuality,
   and Power   104
   Jean Baker Miller

7	Power and Effectiveness: Envisioning an Alternate Paradigm *Maureen Walker*	123
8	Telling the Truth About Power *Jean Baker Miller*	139

SECTION THREE: RCT AND SOCIAL JUSTICE

	Introduction to Section Three: RCT and Social Justice	157
9	Relational-Cultural Practice: Working in a Nonrelational World *Linda Hartling* *Elizabeth Sparks*	158
10	Learning at the Margin: New Models of Strength *Judith V. Jordan*	182
11	Valuing Vulnerability: New Definitions of Courage *Judith V. Jordan*	202
12	Commitment to Connection in a Culture of Fear *Judith V. Jordan*	227
	Index	247

INTRODUCTION

Recent Developments in Relational-Cultural Theory

Judith V. Jordan

In 1976 Jean Baker Miller wrote *Toward a New Psychology of Women*, a groundbreaking book that documented the ways in which women's reality was not being represented in traditional psychological theories. She also pointed to the power of context, the importance of socio-political forces in shaping human development, and the centrality of relationships in women's lives. The book further began to consider the ways in which women's strengths were viewed as weaknesses.

In 1978 a group of four women began meeting to discuss the ways in which the psychology of women continued to mis-represent women's experience. Jean Baker Miller was at the core of this group; she was joined by Irene Stiver, Judith Jordan and Janet Surrey. This group found an institutional home at the Stone Center of Wellesley College when Jean was appointed its first director in 1981. And in 1995 The Jean Baker Miller Training Institute was formed to develop the theory building and developmental/clinical aspects of this work. Since 1981, we

---

Judith V. Jordan, PhD, Jean Baker Miller Training Institute, Harvard Medical School.

have collectively written over 100 "Works in Progress" and produced five core theory books along with many books written by colleagues affiliated with us (see index for list of works in progress and books).

The core ideas of what is now called the Relational-Cultural Theory are that women (although increasingly we think, all people) grow through and toward connection. A model of human development that posits we move from dependence to autonomy does not accurately represent human experience. Furthermore we have questioned the accuracy of a "separate self" paradigm for human development. The metaphor of a separate self suggests that we get stronger and healthier by building firm boundaries, being more independent and that power over others is what leads to a sense of safety or well-being. We suggest that we all need relationships throughout the lifespan and that it is through building good connections that we achieve a sense of well-being and safety. Jean Baker Miller explicitly talked about "growth fostering" relationships as those relationships which create "five good things":

1. a sense of zest
2. clarity about oneself, the other and the relationship
3. a sense of personal worth
4. the capacity to be creative and productive
5. the desire for more connection.

Growth fostering relationships are also characterized by mutual empowerment and mutual empathy. Thus the concept of mutuality and mutual growth takes us away from the model of self-development, which keeps us focused on ways to internalize strengths, become more independent, and develop a "good," independent self. RCT suggests instead that we grow by building growth fostering relationships and community. We grow through and toward relationships.

In such relationships, disconnections will always occur. Empathic failures are ubiquitous in all relationships. If the disconnection can be addressed, however, stronger connections result. For instance, if the less powerful person can state the disconnection and bring attention to the pain caused by a more powerful person and the more powerful person listens empathically and is responsive, the less powerful person learns that she matters, that she can be relationally effective and can bring about positive change in a relationship. If, however, the more powerful person does not listen, responds with invalidation, humiliation or violence, the less powerful person learns to keep that aspect of his or her experience out of relationship. He or she ceases representing herself or himself fully in that relationship. With that often necessary self-protection, the relationship is weakened, mutuality is lessened and people often move into more chronic disconnection. This kind of chronic disconnection is frequent in cases of child neglect or abuse. The child is shut down and the opposite of "the five good things" happens. There is:

1. a drop in energy
2. decreased sense of worth
3. less clarity and more confusion
4. less productivity
5. withdrawal from all relationships.

When people show up for therapy we often see the depression, confusion and withdrawal caused by these conditions.

RCT also makes explicit the ways in which power dynamics in the culture as well as in the family affect people's well-being. Disconnections occur at the societal level when there is a stratification of differences and when the group at the center denigrates and shames the groups at the margin. People are silenced, isolated and shamed as a way of exercising power over them and weakening the representation of their reality in the dominant discourse. People are politically and personally injured by these dynamics. There is a tendency of traditional psychology to over-personalize the problems that people have. Emphasis is put on personal frailty rather than challenging the social conditions that create: rampant abuse of children; stereotyping of people of color and differing sexual orientations; race and class biases that prevent legitimate inclusion in pathways to social movement. The myth of meritocracy is kept alive in such a way that people who "fail" are personally accountable and those that thrive are seen as accomplished, hardworking or sometimes heroic. The invisible and unearned privilege that supports the dominant groups in any culture is kept invisible.

In this volume we present some of the most recent work of the Jean Baker Miller Training Institute (formerly called the Stone Center Theory group). These articles address both therapeutic applications of RCT and present our most recent thinking on the place of power, race, and culture in people's development.

Jean Baker Miller was involved in the early discussion about this volume devoted to relational-cultural theory. She was honored to accept Ellyn Kashak's invitation to develop this issue (book). Although Jean was already quite ill with advanced emphysema at that time, she actively participated in choosing which writings would be included and gave the project her blessing before she passed it on to me. Sadly, her health continued to fail and she died July 29, 2006 before the completion of this project.

Her death has been a great loss for those of us who were fortunate enough to have been her colleague or friend; it was a loss for feminists all over the world. Jean brought a profound vision to the study of the psychology of women. She saw strengths in women where others saw weakness or pathology. Early on, she saw the danger of trying to make women be more like men. In placing power dynamics at the center of her understanding of relationships, she also challenged psychology to move from an overly personalized, decontextualized and supposedly apolitical enterprise to one that publicly accepted its biases and values. She looked at the ways in which the personal and political were inextricably entwined and suggested that psychology embrace that complicated mix in the service of social as well as personal change.

Jean Baker Miller paved the way to a better, more accurate understanding of women's development. But she also believed that social change and social justice had to be part of any responsible model of human development. She was particularly concerned with the disconnections and suffering caused by stratification, marginalization and the exercise of dominance by one group over another. Jean's legacy is a richly elaborated psychology of connection and disconnection. Her clarity and ability to move beyond traditional and limiting paradigms is noteworthy, but her greatest contribution is her challenge to us to create social justice by paying attention to the power of mutual respect and mutual learning in ongoing growth-fostering relationships. Jean Baker Miller reminded us of the profound yearnings of human beings for connection and the desire to participate in the growth of others; she also appreciated the importance of creating and protecting communities of possibility and hope for all people. This volume is dedicated, with love and tremendous gratitude, to Jean Baker Miller, visionary pragmatist, courageous feminist, friend and mentor.

SECTION ONE: RCT AND THERAPY

Introduction to Section One: RCT and Therapy

Section One of this volume looks at the application of Relational-Cultural theory (RCT) to the practice of psychotherapy. The first article by Stiver, Rosen, Surrey and Miller looks at the occasions in therapy when something new and growth-fostering occurs. Eldridge, Surrey, Rosen and Miller then look at the way in which therapists facilitate the capacity to move and be moved by the other. Change entails experiencing a greater freedom of relational movement. In "Strengthening Resilience in a Risky World," Hartling reviews the literature describing individual, internal characteristics associated with resilience and explores the relational aspects of these characteristics. In Walker's chapter, "When Racism gets Personal: Toward Relational Healing," we see the ways in which racial anxiety impedes movement toward authenticity, mutuality and empowerment in intimate relationships Walker notes that the anxieties endemic to race-based culture have the potential to thwart our most earnest efforts to make and maintain good connection. In "How Therapy Helps When the Culture Hurts," Walker examines the impact of cultural disconnections on the therapy relationship.

Creative Moments
in Relational-Cultural Therapy

Irene Pierce Stiver
Wendy Rosen
Janet Surrey
Jean Baker Miller

SUMMARY. Creative moments in therapy are those occasions when something new and growth-fostering occurs. This article offers three illustrations and a discussion of these characteristics. It is based on a panel

---

Irene Pierce Stiver, PhD, was Lecturer in Psychiatry at Harvard Medical School, Director Emerita of the Psychology Department at McLean Hospital, Belmont, MA and Faculty Scholar of the Jean Baker Miller Training Institute; Co-author of *Women's Growth in Connection* and *The Healing Connection*. Dr. Stiver died on September 24, 2000.

Wendy Rosen, PhD, LICSW, is Attending Supervisor at Mclean Hospital and maintains a private practice of psychotherapy and supervision in Cambridge, MA. She is a contributing author of *Women's Growth in Diversity*.

Janet Surrey, PhD, is Founding Scholar and Faculty, JBMTI; Attending Psychologist McLean Hospital/Harvard Medical School; co-editor of *Mothering Against the Odds* and co-author of *Women's Growth in Connection* and *We Have to Talk: Healing Dialogues Between Women and Men*.

Jean Baker Miller, MD (1927-2006), was Founding Scholar and Director of the Jean Baker Miller Training Institute at the Stone Center, Wellesley College; Clinical Professor of Psychiatry at Boston University School of Medicine; author of *Toward a New Psychology of Women*; and co-author of *The Healing Connection* and *Women's Growth in Connection*. She was a practicing psychiatrist and psychoanalyst.

discussion held at the Stone Center-Harvard Medical School/Cambridge Hospital "Learning from Women Conference" in April, 2000.

INTRODUCTION

What do we mean by *creative moments*? We will discuss the meanings of these moments at greater length after presenting a few examples. However, as an initial suggestion, we will say that creative moments refers to those times in therapy when something new happens–something is created. From the perspective of Relational-Cultural Theory, they are the occasions when the new creation is growth-fostering, that is, it propels the relationship in a healing and enlarging direction. They lead to what we call "movement-in-relationship." The relationship deepens and expands and so do each (or all) of the participants.

VIGNETTE ONE: "SUSAN"

By Irene P. Stiver, PhD

I will be talking about my work with a woman in her fifties whom I'll call Susan. She entered therapy one day with a sense of urgency; even before she sat down she started talking. She began with, "I've been wanting to ask you for some time, what do you think of all this Clinton business?" This was the beginning of the Kenneth Starr revelations, with Monica's confirmation that she had had "a relationship with the President"; there were loud accusations of perjury and predictions that this would lead to the President's impeachment.

Various thoughts, some desperate, went quickly through my mind. How could I tell her how I really felt? My feelings were very strong, if complicated, about this whole business, and I knew that our politics would not be similar.

She came from a very steadfast Republican family. At the same time, I knew that one of our major themes in therapy was her mother's silence and its profound effect on her. She never knew what her mother thought of anything. As a child, if she tried to pursue her mother about what she wanted, thought, or would do, her mother would convey non-verbally (by facial and bodily expression) that she experienced Susan as too aggressive and forceful; she wanted Susan to back off.

Susan had recently started to date a man for the first time since her divorce more than five years ago and with great trepidation had introduced him to her parents. She told me her father said, "He seems very nice." I then asked what her mother thought of him and she said she had no idea. Her mother had said nothing.

When I wondered if she considered asking her mother what she thought, she looked really horrified and said it made her anxious to even contemplate that possibility. She felt it would be an assault on her mother. Her mother would not be able to tolerate such an assault, and Susan would end up feeling like a bad person.

This story and others like it flashed through my mind in the short period while she was framing the question, and I was trying to determine what to do. I felt I *had* to answer. I could not replicate this part of her relationship with her mother, that is, evade and not appreciate her *need to know* and all that meant. So I said, "Well I must admit, I am angry at everyone involved but I am especially infuriated with Starr who has his own agenda, that is, he is out to get Clinton. I think Clinton was very irresponsible and so was Monica."

Susan listened and then asked more about what I thought of Clinton "getting away with" perjury and what message that sent to the country. Her new boyfriend had said now all drug users can lie about taking drugs because the President committed perjury; they will think that they can get away with it. I then said something–with thoughts of Carol Gilligan–about how moral issues can be seen in context and I thought that when a married man is having an affair, especially if he's President, he would typically lie about it. I did not think it was of the same order as other perjuries. We were at this point having a conversation with a give and take between us.

She then asked me how my feminist colleagues and I felt about Clinton's affair with Monica. He had betrayed his wife and was taking advantage of a very young woman, an intern in the White House. I said my sense was that feminists were mixed in their reactions. I had read other perspectives and discussed this with other women and they clearly had differences of opinion. That his behavior was outrageous was the general consensus–for me as well.

But another consideration I and some other feminists had was that Clinton had really done a great deal for women, more than any other president in terms of his stand on certain issues and the appointments he made. Even though he treated his wife terribly with his affairs and sexual betrayals, he also seemed to truly value Hillary for her intelligence and strength, more than other presidents and their wives.

All the time I was talking, I was thinking, "Oh my God. What am I doing? How will this affect the relationship–the transference?" So I said, "You know, to share these ideas goes against much of my background as a therapist; that is, a therapist should not bring her personal opinions into the therapy; it would have a negative impact on the therapy and on her. I am concerned that this might get in the way of the work we are doing."

She responded with much energy, saying how important it was to her that I had been *immediately* responsive. She said that it took so much courage for her to ask me and it would have felt awful if I had not responded. She had come in with a sense of urgency but *had not dared to think* of how I might respond.

After the session, I was very distressed since I still worried that I had done something wrong. I feared that I might have silenced and suppressed her ability to hold on and express opinions different from mine. After all, I had more power to influence her and there was the danger she would feel ashamed for having a different perspective. I thought I should have explored the many complicated meanings these questions had for her and somehow found a way to be less definitive about how I felt.

But I also knew that what I did was more syntonic with our Relational-Cultural Model and my understanding of Susan. So despite my doubts and concerns about what I had done, I was strongly influenced by our concepts about reframing therapy. First, to address the transference issue, we have said that we did not agree with the notion that the therapist's neutrality was essential to the development of the transference. Instead, we believe that: (1) transference develops under all circumstances and (2) as long as the therapist remains relatively neutral she may not perceive the significant differences between this new relationship with her therapist and those relational images from the past that the patient brings into therapy.

In contrast, when the therapist is able to create a new relational context that is mutually empathic and empowering, she will provide a fertile ground for the patient to develop more positive relational images and their meanings. I felt I had to provide her with a different relational context from her experience at home, a context in which her curiosity could be respected and responded to.

Thus, our understanding of the goal of therapy had to lead me to respond as I had, that is, to create a mutually empathic and mutually empowering relationship so that the patient can feel safe enough over time to represent herself more fully. To engage with her in this mutually empathic way, I had to be authentic and deeply appreciative of her sense of urgency and her need to know what I thought. I was moved by the courage it took for her to take such a risk with me. She risked that I would confirm the dangers of asking such a personal question and that I would humiliate her and cut her off by refusing to be responsive to what she was asking of me. I believe that *she was* moved by my willingness to share both my vulnerability and concerns in the process.

However, after the session I continued to obsess and worry despite my awareness of what I've just said. It is still amazing to me after all the years of doing this work and my deep belief and commitment to these ideas, that all the authority figures from my past can still lead me to doubt what I truly *know*.

I dreaded my next session with Susan, but my dread quickly dissipated in seeing her mood and presence when she arrived. She began by telling me how important it was that I had respected her question, and what it meant to have someone see her questions and curiosity as justified. She talked about never having dared to ask questions like that of anyone, feeling sure they would not like it.

Later in this and subsequent sessions, she spoke about realizing how judgmental a person she was and thought that our discussion had helped her see that more clearly. Indeed, she was very judgmental, especially of herself. She went back to a time when she learned that a woman teacher in one of her children's schools was having an affair with a male teacher. She was scandalized and wanted to "report it" but she didn't. And now she could tell me about an analogous situation in her own life many years ago–a secret affair, which filled her with enormous guilt and scorn toward herself. It was a new revelation and a new awareness.

This creative moment occurred about a year-and-a-half ago. Susan is braver now in daring to confront and ask people what they think, and our relationship continues to grow with all the expected glitches and disconnections en route.

VIGNETTE TWO: "MAURA"

By Wendy Rosen, PhD, LICSW

I had known Maura for about three months as her couples therapist. She and her partner eventually went their separate ways, which at the time saddened me very much. Even though I'd held no illusions about the sustaining power of their relationship, I just liked them both so much and I wished that each of them could find and keep love. At Maura's request, I referred her partner for individual therapy, and they both saw me through the break up. Following termination, Maura chose not to continue any therapy, and I didn't hear from either of them for almost two years.

Maura had always struck me as a very passionate, powerful, and absolutely compelling woman. She was sharp, wise, ambitious, incredibly street-smart, and verbally formidable on the outside but she also held certain other parts of herself within a very protected place. Maura revealed these aspects of herself much more sparingly, entrusting what has proven to be a very big and very fragile heart to a select few. That's one of the reasons why this break up had been so painful for her. It had been a very long time since she had allowed herself to open up to someone again, having been crushed several years prior by the loss of a woman with whom she had been deeply in love.

When Maura left couples therapy with me, she had also left her mark on me. I don't think I could have articulated it at the time, but it had something to do with what I experienced as her deep sensitivity, her courage, and her tremendous generosity. She inspired me in some unusual way, and I felt privileged in her trust of me. I knew I would miss Maura and with her departure, I felt my own painful sense of remorse for the loss she was left to carry with her.

Maura's life had been a series of tough challenges. She was the oldest child growing up in a large, extended, close-knit Irish Catholic family. Both her parents were from very large, struggling, working-class families, and they had married young. Her mother, whose family had been quite poor and who'd had a particularly rough life of her own, was perpetually overwhelmed, anxious, short-tempered, and physically abusive, primarily to Maura. She always perceived Maura as the toughest and most durable of her children, and thus, never spared the rod on her. Maura quickly learned to be tough. Her father made it clear early on that she would have to fight her own fights, both literally and figuratively. He was a rugged, no-nonsense kind of guy who repeatedly emphasized the importance of family bonds and loyalty, until one day when, with no explanation, he abruptly left his wife and children for another woman.

This was devastating to his family, but particularly to Maura, who felt betrayed in some fundamental way. Here was a man who had consistently espoused the creed that "family is everything" and then turned around and walked out on his own. This stood as a glaring and wrenching hypocrisy in the face of Maura's, by then, strong personal ethos. Given her mother's emotional fragility and relative inability to fight for the protection of her children, especially now that she was on her own, Maura felt extraordinarily responsible for her family, particularly for three of her four younger siblings.

Maura was extremely close to her sister, Kathleen, who was closest in age to her. Kathleen knew Maura better than most, and she had a remarkably generous spirit. Everyone loved Kathleen, but especially Maura. If Maura was the one to whom everyone turned for strength and material support, Kathleen was the one to whom Maura turned for essential moral support. In Maura's eyes, Kathleen was the real beating heart of the family.

When Maura was a child, she had serious learning disabilities, which often left her feeling humiliated and ashamed in school. She compensated for these challenges through her considerable physical prowess and tremendous athletic capabilities. She engaged in numerous sports and became a competitive athlete. Never one to fold in the face of challenge, Maura devoted herself to competing and winning, refusing ever to become, in her words, a "cupcake." A cupcake was soft in the middle, and thus, would inevitably "choke" when called upon to enter the real contest in both sport and life.

Succumbing to pain or hardship in any form was simply not an option, and any feelings that set Maura off course were to be quickly eradicated. Maura's oft-repeated mantra was "buck up." Despite an academic history marred by extraordinary challenges, Maura managed to get athletic scholarships, graduate, and continue her athletic competition, in addition to some coaching. She attracted a lot of interest from others as a result of her strength, courage, and shrewd savvy. She knew how to survive, how to win, and above all, how to get people moving and go for the best deal. Many of Maura's most enduring connections were forged at the negotiating table. If you were willing to come to that table, she would always meet you there, and no one would ever leave it without having gained something. One of her most famous and engaging lines has always been, "Come on! Work with me here!" And most everyone did. This has since led her to a very successful life in business.

After Maura terminated her couples work with me, I would periodically hear random bits of news of her through the grapevine of people we remotely knew in common. I always felt a surge of warmth at these moments and was happy to have even small scraps of information about how she was managing post-breakup. She'd left a lasting impression on me, and I always hoped she would find happiness in a relationship with someone who could really appreciate her in all of her unique complexity.

One of the more significant events that I heard about proved to be both painful and rather complicated. One of Maura's younger siblings, a sister, was found to be having a serious substance abuse problem and was increasingly unable to care for her very young daughter, Cara. Given that there was no father in the picture and that neither Maura's mother or her other siblings were in any kind of favorable position to pitch in, Maura quickly took over. This was so much her way. If a problem presented itself and Maura could do something about it, she did, with no questions asked and not a moment's hesitation. Cara, four years old, moved in with Maura, and suddenly her life was irrevocably changed.

Motherhood, of any sort, had never been a part of Maura's vision for herself. She was single, gay, and on a fast-paced business track, always entertaining interesting new entrepreneurial opportunities. She had a number of friends, most of them without children. Her rapid trajectory came to a screeching halt, necessitating a complete revamping of present and future plans. While she adored Cara and had no question about the validity of her decision, Maura also faced some very real personal loss with this change in her life. Her responsibility for the caretaking of Cara had now become her primary commitment, rendering her other ambitions and way of life very much secondary. Not one to indulge grief excessively, Maura didn't miss a beat in transitioning to her new role. She once told me in no uncertain terms, "I will never spend time wanting what I can't have."

About a year or so after Maura became Cara's legal guardian, I heard another piece of news. Around this time, her closest sister and veritable soul mate, Kathleen, was visiting them. They'd been having a great weekend together, until Sunday morning, when Maura went in to awaken Kathleen and found her dead. Kathleen had had a longstanding heart condition and suffered a heart attack during the night.

Maura was completely devastated. In her typical, responsible way, she practically single-handedly took care of all the necessary arrangements, culminating in a very moving and heavily attended funeral. Kathleen was well-loved by many people.

When I heard the news, which was not long after Kathleen's death, I was stunned and, quite simply, utterly grief-stricken for Maura. I immediately felt the array of emotional implications for her, knowing full well the weight she was already under. Her life just seemed to be punctuated by a string of significant, often wrenching losses to which she responded with a renewed commitment to courage, but also, with a little less faith and hope and just a little more feeling of aching solitude each and every time.

I decided to call her. Even though it had been at least two years since we had seen one another and although I had heard this recent news via a rather circuitous network, I had little question about my decision to call. Once again, I felt another of Maura's devastating losses. In my remorse about the loss of her partner in our couples therapy, I now faced an opportunity to meet up once again with her grief. I still had the desire and the need to try and meet her there for whatever it was worth.

Maura was surprised to hear from me, but we spent no time at all catching up. Neither one of us seemed to require it. Rather, I shared with her my deep sorrow regarding the death of her sister, and she moved seamlessly into sharing with me the abyss of her grief. The word she most often used to describe it was "brutal." I recently looked this up in the dictionary, and its definition was "cruel, merciless." She couldn't have put it more aptly.

When Maura allowed herself to attach, to really love, she entrusted her whole heart to that relationship. To lose the relationship became for her an act of almost physical cruelty, an action completely without mercy. Maura experienced her life as anything but filled with acts of mercy. She learned all too early that she would have to fight all her own fights and that asking for help was out of the question. During our conversation, I asked Maura if there was anything I could do to be of help to her. I asked her if it might be useful to just come in and talk, and then, without even thinking about it, I offered to meet her somewhere else if she wanted, perhaps simply to talk over a cup of coffee. She paused for a moment and then responded that she didn't really feel the need for any kind of therapy but that she thought it would feel good to meet with me over a cup of tea. We made plans to see one another in a few days at a deli near my office.

Maura and I met twice at the deli, each time with her insisting on buying me lunch and acknowledging gratitude for my spending this time with her. She shared with me the detailed circumstances of Kathleen's death, her relentless and unbearable grief complete with an array of physical and stress-related symptoms, the terrible saga of her other sister's tragic substance abuse problems, and the care of her niece, Cara. Maura was suffering badly, and I wanted to try and be there for her in the ways that I could. At the end of our second lunch together, I suggested to her that we might think about meeting together in my office where we'd have more privacy and where I could perhaps help her through what was clearly a most devastating time in her life. We agreed that there needn't be a commitment to anything ongoing, unless she chose it.

Since that time, Maura has asked to see me twice a week and has allowed me access to a little more of her heart each and every time, while without realizing it, she already had found a permanent place in mine.

Not too long ago, Maura told me a story about her endless array of organized outings with Cara and a whole group of her little friends from school and Girl Scouts. She is forever planning fun activities, often of the athletic type, including biking, swimming, softball, skating, and skiing, to name a few, all followed by ice cream. Needless to say, the girls thrill to these events. Often, they excitedly shout out to her, "Maura, what are we doing today?" Each time this occurs, she turns to them and answers, "Girls, take out your memory books. Today we are making another great memory."

VIGNETTE THREE: "KIRK"

By Janet Surrey, PhD

Most change and movement in therapy feels gradual, winding in and out, back and forth, but this was one of those exceptional moments–powerful, instantaneous, and unforgettable. Although rare, it is the kind of moment that keeps us alive, keeps us "keeping on," and gives depth and meaning to this difficult work. For Kirk, the client with whom I shared this moment, it was pivotal and transformative.

Kirk actually asked me many times to find a way to speak or write about his therapy. He wanted me to give his name and saw no reason for confidentiality. As a journalist, he felt something important like this ought to be reported. As you will see, this was quite a distance from where we began.

Kirk originally came to see me at the age of 46, in the context of the break up of his second marriage. As a last resort, his wife had asked him to see a relational therapist. In the first session, he described himself as a "recovering white male. I've benefited from every privilege; I'm white, male, affluent, educated, and tall. I don't have any right to be here. You're wasting your time." He was, as you can hear, sardonic, sarcastic, and very skeptical about this first experience of therapy. Kirk was a successful newspaper editor, political commentator, and activist. He was a rising star in his work but felt little gratification or joy in it and little sense of worth.

In his relationships with women and with his three young children, he felt enormous shame and deficiency: a "true failure." This was what he felt was most true about himself; that "something is just missing." Kirk was chronically, not clinically, depressed, emotionally constricted, very judgmental, bristly, and quick to anger. He used his wry humor to maintain distance and control and to cut off any hint of emotional joining, any possibility of holding a connection or surrendering to the relational moment where something new can happen.

Kirk felt responsible for the difficulties in his marriages. He knew he was unable to accept vulnerability or empathize with others, particularly women. He recognized his unwillingness and awkwardness in showing any depth of feeling except anger or disdain. This was part of his success as a political analyst: his incisive and biting humor coupled with great intelligence. At first quite hostile, he began to soften. The anger turned to teasing. We laughed a lot together as this was his primary way of connecting.

Kirk knew of my gender dialogue work and my interest in male-female relationships and frequently he would say to me: "Hey, I'm a man, what can you expect?"

In the first year of our work together, I listened to his story and began to feel some empathy. He desperately wanted me to help him learn to be a father. We talked in the greatest detail about his children, in the process building interest, curiosity, understanding, and connection. Through this conversation, he began to touch on his own sadness and loneliness as a young boy, growing up in an isolated rural area as an only child. His mother was diabetic and from the time he was eight her health deteriorated; she eventually became totally blind and bedridden. She died when he was 22. While she was alive, his mother never left the house and he remembered coming home from school everyday and sitting with her telling her all about his day. He felt he had to be "her light" and bring interesting news from the outside world. But they could never acknowledge together any of the difficult feelings of grief or loss.

His father was a good and reliable caretaker, but also could not express or share his emotions. Even in talking about the past, Kirk continued to avoid any relational connection that might evoke his sadness. We wondered what it was like for his mother and imagined that she tried to protect him from her grief. He imagined that he too might have been trying to protect her, as well as himself, by staying away from his painful feelings.

Weekly sessions with Kirk were difficult and not something I looked forward to. I often felt frustrated and exhausted and had to work extremely hard to maintain any emotional connection or relational continuity. Although I knew some part of him desired connection, his relational "dread" as described by Stephen Bergman (1990) and his strategies of disconnection–humor, anger, sarcasm, and especially self-denigration–were well developed and very controlling. I found myself empathizing with the women in his life; the gender issues were always present between us. Kirk began to be curious about me and my work and about therapy. He began to understand that he was not simply "empty" and not simply afraid of feeling his sadness and loneliness–but was more afraid of feeling alone with them. He had no experience of or images of relationships where feelings moved between and connected people. He did have images of relationships where feelings of vulnerability were associated with humiliation (part of male socialization in an all boys private school) and also of relationships where any emotional exposure led to feelings of shame and deficiency.

One year into therapy, Kirk was at a routine medical appointment to investigate a chronic cough and was diagnosed with fast-growing metastatic lung cancer. He lived for 13 months after this diagnosis. I remember that he called me between sessions to tell me this news. I remember that when he came in the next time, I changed my seat and moved from a chair further away to sit right next to him. I was startled to observe how much more open and willing to be with him I was in the face of illness and possible death. What a lesson about my own personal and professional strategies of disconnection!

At first Kirk's bitterness, anger, sense of loss of a future, and particularly his mourning the chance to grow were stunning. He struggled against his own depression and resignation. And then he began to work earnestly on trying to be open and present to complete the work he needed to do in all his relationships. Often he felt empty, blocked, and helpless to change. I referred him for bodywork, to a men's cancer support group, and to a meditation group. We began to start our sessions with silence. He began to talk about his life as a mosaic of moments with each moment having its own completeness and beauty.

Halfway through his last year, as he became physically symptomatic, he asked me in one session to work with him on a visualization exercise. He was trying to locate a safe, peaceful, psychological place where he could find refuge; a place to go in the face of fear and pain and ultimately, as I look back, in the face of death. He was describing a scene close to his childhood home, actually very close to where I grew up. I felt very connected to the scene that he described as sitting on a porch of an old abandoned house, looking out at a soft green meadow, listening to the sound of a running brook in the background. I said to Kirk, probably with some frustration, but mostly I believe wistful sadness and hard-won acceptance: "I'm still not sure if you want me or anyone else there *with you*."

Although I had been speaking to this particular scene, I realized this touched a core question for him.

He stopped and answered softly with feeling, "I'm not sure either."

He was clear, direct, authentic, at one with his thoughts and words in the relationship.

We sat in silence. I sensed something happening. Finally, he looked at me with tears, and said, "I can feel how hard it is for you–when you're trying to be with me and I don't know what I want."

Another silence. I began to worry about whether I had revealed too much of myself. I felt doubt and shame about his focus on how hard it was for me, that maybe I had expressed too much of my own painful struggles in relationships with men. But the meaning for him was obviously too significant, and I did not let my therapist strategies of disconnection–especially of turning the focus back on him–get in the way of letting him be with me.

He began to talk about feeling something grow between us. He noticed that he could just stay with my pain without taking it back to how it reflected on him, on how he had failed again. He described a feeling of love and compassion for me–for women, feeling women's struggle to relate to him–to men.

He then described feeling a sense of expansiveness and buoyancy and feeling a new energy surging through his body, particularly through his hands.

Our eyes met and he held the gaze with me for some time, both of us tearful but smiling. I knew we both felt a deep appreciation for where we had been and where we now were. This "seeing together," this understanding reverberated between us. How difficult to describe mutual empathy, relational power, the five good things–healing connection, zest, spirit, interbeing, relational being, I and Thou, We.

After that, Kirk described in his life a growing capacity to be with others, which brought him great joy. He let friends be with him in new ways as he died, although some important relationships remained very difficult and unmoving.

Our relationship remained immensely important to both of us and I saw him up to the day before his death. I promised him I would share his experience although I have not yet found a reporter who wanted to write this story for his newspaper.

I have pondered the memory of this moment many, many times. It still remains a mystery, an experience of hard work *and* grace. As a therapist, it was not so much what I did but what I knew *not* to do in that moment and where I was willing to go with him, where we could go together. We came to this very alive moment of healing connection, of mutual presence together. Daniel Stern calls this a "now" moment. Clearly this moment grew out of all the moments before and of the new relational experiences and relational images growing over time. Its meaning was heightened by the closeness of death, which moved both of us beyond our protective and habitual strategies of disconnection. Facing death can help us drop the past and drop the projection of past wounds onto the future. Connection is always in the present, this present moment.

A relational moment like this contains and expresses in microcosm the *whole* relationship. Its texture was built on shared experience, understanding, trust, and love. The moment was deeply moving for each of us, changing both–differently but deeply shared. Through the work of weaving authentic and empathic connections between us, we also touched the dimension of the larger cultural disconnection and the struggle for mutual relationship between men and women–"stepping out" of patriarchy, as Carol Gilligan would say. Both of us were deeply aware of the larger gendered meaning of the moment. Coming to this moment of mutuality through the particulars of who we are, therapist-client, woman-man, through history, through culture, touching into our deeply human connection.

Finally, this moment had a timeless dimension. It remains still very alive, mysterious, vivid, and limitless in its truth. I feel Kirk's presence absolutely with me as I speak of this today, even though it occurred nearly eight years ago. And I carry this moment–this We–as a resource, a place of faith, resilience, and power into my encounters in therapy and in life.

DISCUSSION

By Jean Baker Miller, MD

What any therapist would call a creative moment will depend on her theory of therapy. As we see, these moments reflect some of the major tenets of Relational-Cultural Theory. That theory rests on the belief that the essence of living and developing is connecting in a way that fosters growth. This reaching for connection represents people's basic motivation, yearning, desire. Growth-fostering connections are defined by the fact that they lead to some or all of what we've called "the five good things," i.e., a sense of increased energy or zest, an increased motivation and ability to take action, greater understanding of self, other, and the relationship, increased sense of worth, and a greater desire for more connection (Miller, 1988; Miller & Stiver, 1997).

THEORY OF THERAPY

However, all of us inevitably experience disconnections, especially as we live in an overall society in which any one group of people has more power over another. These "power-over" conditions reach in to affect us even in our most personal childhood and adult relationships. In times of disconnection, we experience the reverse of "the five good things" and also several additional negative consequences, especially a sense of psychological isolation.

This sense of isolation is devastating and so threatens a child's (or adult's) sense of psychological integrity that s/he will do everything possible to try to avoid it. What people do is: keep parts of their important experience out of their relationships–the thoughts and feelings that seem impossible to bring into connection. Thus, over time, people learn to keep parts of themselves out of connection in order to try to make connections. We see this as the *central relational paradox* and also the fundamental idea guiding therapy (Miller, 1988; Miller & Stiver, 1997).

In therapy, the path to healing is connecting and this connecting is based on a particular form of mutual empathy (Jordan, Kaplan, Miller, Stiver, & Surrey, 1991). That is, the therapist must be able to feel with the patient's experience–at least to a large extent; and the patient must feel the therapist feeling with her (Miller & Stiver, 1997). We see this illustrated in the examples here. Jan's example especially highlights this point. Sometimes in creative moments, a person can feel another person feeling with her or with an aspect of her experience in a way that hadn't crystallized for her ever before.

Mutual empathy leads to the "five good things," and they are the major components of mutual empowerment (Miller, 1988; Miller & Stiver, 1997). An especially powerful part of mutual empowerment in therapy is that the patient can see that she has had an impact on the therapist. Feeling this impact is vitally important because in serious disconnections a person has often felt that she could not really reach or affect the other person(s). This is another way of saying that she has felt powerless (Miller & Stiver, 1997). In these creative moments, we see that it is not an impact in some general sense; it is a person's feeling that her feelings and thoughts *matter* to the other person. They are *heard* and *felt* and they matter just because she has felt them. We can see this in all of the examples.

When people feel that their thoughts and feelings don't matter to others, they resort to many other methods of trying to have an impact. These methods are usually coercive and distancing of other people, for example, what we call passive-aggressive behavior. There are many others.

SOME CHARACTERISTICS OF CREATIVE MOMENTS

Creative moments are many and varied, large and small. I will mention here only a few of their characteristics. In some moments, the therapist may find herself outside of her accustomed "comfort zone." She has to expand her repertoire, which usually means she has to take a risk, move into the unfamiliar. She opens herself to new experience and potentially new emotional and cognitive learning. Doing so often leads her to feelings of vulnerability and self-doubt. All of the panelists describe these experiences.

Even as she feels vulnerable, the therapist chooses to be true to the integrity of the relationship. To behave in a more formulaic mode could violate the experience patient and therapist have had together. If the therapist betrayed the experience of the relationship, she could cause a serious disconnection. So, for example, if Irene had not answered Susan's question, Susan could have felt that Irene was betraying all that Irene had seemed to understand about how devastating it was for her when her mother was unresponsive. They had talked together about how Susan felt so totally obliterated at these times, so isolated and so helpless.

This integrity rests on a basis of mutual empathy. The therapist has a sense that her actions emerge from her empathic understanding of her patient. She also has a sense of how her patient will respond. Most importantly, she has a sense of how ready her patient may be to move into new experience. Likewise, the therapist has a sense of the level of mutual empathy in the relationship, that is, thoughts and feelings about how much she and her patient share an understanding of their relationship and also how empathic her patient is with her (the therapist's) feelings and intent. Of course, the therapist's perception of the level of mutual empathy in the relationship is never perfect or total.

In these moments, we usually see the therapist allowing herself to be more open and authentic (Miller, Jordan, Stiver, Walker, Surrey, & Eldridge, 1999). She is more "present" as opposed to withholding. Allowing herself to be more vulnerable in all these ways means that the therapist is willing to relinquish some of her power and control, that is, she does not stay within the traditional methods by which therapists tend to maintain control. Notice how much less in control Irene felt than if she had said something like, "I wonder why you ask?"

This willingness to move toward less power in therapy does not ever mean relinquishing responsibility. The two have been easily confused. The therapist is always responsible for working toward the goal of therapy, which is to benefit the patient. While therapists must be responsible, we have been led to believe that this must mean using power and control over the patient. I believe this confusion follows from our basic cultural concepts, which readily elude responsibility and control. It rests on a lack of faith in relationship and in the belief that the therapist's authenticity and caring can lead to the kind of connection that will be beneficial for the patient.

Because of their interchange, Susan was able to say to Irene, "It took so much courage for me to ask you and it would have felt awful if you had not responded." It was very meaningful that Susan could say this. If Irene hadn't responded as she did and Susan had felt awful, Susan may not have been able to say that. Then this feeling could have become a troublesome, hidden, unexpressed factor in their relationship.

Traditionally, therapists would say that Irene's actions would prevent Susan from getting to more underlying and important issues. Instead, we see that Irene's recognition of the integrity of their relationship and her willingness to be authentic and vulnerable led to Susan's ability to reveal more, not less. She can talk about the very central issue of unresponsiveness and also about her own extra-marital affair. With this, she was able to have less unproductive guilt and scorn for herself. She also saw more of the truth about herself as critical and judgmental.

Wendy, too, was acting with respect for the integrity of her relationship with Maura. Wendy felt that Maura was "paralyzed by grief"; she also knew Maura's whole history of not feeling able to expect responsiveness and her likely inability to express her needs directly. Wendy speaks of her "need to meet Maura in her grief." This, like the features in the other examples, could be seen as some pathological, or, at least, therapeutically inappropriate need of Wendy's or, as we're suggesting, it can be a desire to be true to the integrity of the relationship, to what Wendy and Maura had been through together. This was a conscious choice Wendy made; it was not a compulsion.

STAGES OF THERAPY

We do not mean to suggest that we should go around looking for creative moments. Rather, they emerge when we stay close to what we think and feel are going on in the relational work in therapy. They do not arise out of the blue. Usually a great deal of work has led up to them. However, they can sometimes occur early in therapy. Two years ago, as part of a panel on Therapists' Authenticity at this conference, Maureen Walker presented an example that occurred in a very first session (Miller et al., 1999).

That example illustrates so beautifully all of the features mentioned here and more. Maureen, an African-American woman, was in training and had to take as her patient, John, the next person in rotation. John was a racist, denigrating, white man and from his first words, it was clear that Maureen was not in her "comfort zone." Indeed, no one should have to go through this kind of racist experience. Maureen described how she was tempted to use her power as a therapist to put down this man and to stay out of connection with him. Instead she was able to use her empathy with the small amount she knew about him and "to say something to John about how the decision to talk to me must not have been an easy one." I refer you to the paper for the rest of the story but, in summary, this proved a most creative moment. Both John and Maureen stayed in the therapy, which was a huge accomplishment. Further, Maureen set the stage for the kind of creative and authentic movement-in-relationship that amazingly ensued. A most productive mutual growth occurred over the next two years.

CREATION VERSUS INTERPRETATION

Creative moments are very different from interpretations. One central difference is that they are mutual. Both people tend to be engaged, active, and authentic. This is different from the therapist dispensing insight. An interpretation may sometimes be helpful in aiding a person to understand something about her past, but that is different from the experience of creative change.

This change is not on an intellectual level only, nor even on an intellectual and emotional level. It is relational, which means integrated through several levels, as in "the five good things" explained earlier. And it becomes, therefore, empowering. Again, it's a new creation, a creation of a new experience, something that hadn't existed before in the relationship–and often, something that hadn't existed before ever.

In therapy, as in life, it is the welcoming of the new that is so important. This is often thwarted in the course of development for all of us to varying degrees. In various ways, we all can then become stuck in old paths, either with our strategies of disconnection or our old relational images, as described in several papers (Miller & Stiver, 1994, 1996, 1997). We become anxious, vigilant, guarded, restricted, and the like. Our culture, I believe, leads to these problems, as I'll suggest below.

Instead, in creative moments, we step into new experience, onto the untrodden path, often the frightening untrodden path. And the great thing is, if we find it, it is different, better than the old. The great discovery in terms of Relational-Cultural Therapy is that a person can find that as she brings more of herself into connection, she is reversing the central relational paradox. She is being more herself and also more connected–something that had seemed impossible.

We should probably call these moments "co-creative moments" because they are truly created by two people; in group or family therapy it may be more than two people. They are co-created in the work that leads up to them as well as in the moments, themselves. They may be initiated by the action of the patient or the therapist, for example, in Irene's illustration it was the patient; in Wendy's it was the therapist. However, the essence is that the other person(s) is able to move into the action, to move it forward, something we've called "movement-in-relationship" (Miller & Stiver, 1997).

NEW CONNECTIONS, NEW PERSON

The fact that the patient is a co-creator, a participant, leads to another factor in Relational-Cultural Therapy: the patient finds that *she* can be part of creating connection and she can participate in movement-in-relationship. The patient is finding in herself a creative and connecting force. Why is this important? When we suffer disconnections as children and even as adults, one of the terrible features is that we tend to believe that we are the reason for the disconnection. We then develop the inner construction of ourselves as the bad, even evil, person. This is a terrible sense of oneself as a person who cannot make good connections and thus, cannot make good things happen. We have elaborated on this point in various ways, describing it as "condemned isolation" and as a major source of negative relational images and meanings (Miller, 1988; Miller

& Stiver, 1997) and the source of shame (Jordan, 1989; Hartling, Rosen, Walker, & Jordan, 2000).

When a person begins to experience herself as a person who can make connections, she also begins to see herself as a different kind of person; she can create different relational images and meanings about herself. In these moments, she can often see the contrast between her more restricted and disconnected self and a new way to be.

Kirk, in Jan's example, so poignantly illustrates this point. He moved into connection, with a "feeling of deep connection, love, and empathy" for Jan struggling to be in relationship with him. He saw how hard it was to be with him. He saw a truth about "the old" but in the same moment he could glimpse "the new," saying, "I can just be with you and not take it back to me." This moment illustrates how powerful moving into connection was for him. At the same time, it opened a vision of himself as different, not the old isolated, lonely self, but a person who *can* make connection.

The moment also illustrates mutuality beautifully. While the moment entailed Kirk's movement into connection, empathy, and love, Jan also felt much greater connection with him and with parts of her past experience with men. What each felt was certainly not identical. Each was at a different point but they were connecting profoundly.

While the purpose was not and should never be for Jan's benefit, we can see that such moments always foster the growth of the therapist. When we truly try to examine what goes on in therapy, I think we have to see that such moments of growth are inevitably mutual.

For Susan, too, experiences like these lead to a change in her relational images and thus in her image of herself, away from those of a person whose actions lead to disconnection and away from feeling like a "dangerous, aggressive person." Now she can see a possibility of herself as a person whose initiative leads to a very productive series of connections. Her interest, her desire does not have to mean disconnection and terrible consequences. She was also able to see the possibility of herself as less critical and less judgmental, both in regard to others and to herself.

Maura also could begin to include her desire and her need for responsiveness in her picture of herself. We have not been talking about a person who has lost every sort of connection but the specific kinds of connection that have become problematic in her life. Maura had many connections, but she did not have the kind of connection in which she could be a person with desires and needs and expect others to understand and respond to them.

I am suggesting we can see more than the reversal of the central relational paradox in a non-dynamic way. A person can see herself in the process of *becoming* as opposed to "fixed," stuck. She can see herself becoming more the kind of person she would want to be and had not felt she could be. To feel herself in movement in this way is so different from feeling herself so stuck. To put this another way, I don't think that we find some fixed, hidden "true self." I believe we can move into *becoming* a fuller, stronger person, into movement rather than fixity. And we can include in that person qualities we had not thought possible.

CAUTIONS

As we know, movement in therapy is never a straight line onward and upward. Indeed, after creative moments like these, we often find a person returning to acting in an old disconnected way. We have described this tendency in detail, saying that therapists must honor a person's "strategies of disconnection" (Miller & Stiver, 1994; 1997).

Are there dangers to these creative moments? Yes, there may be. These dangers can occur if the therapist's actions are not well attuned to the specific relationship and well timed to the poignant moment in the relationship. With another person it may not have been at all helpful that Irene, Jan, or Wendy acted in the way they did.

However, we are not always so attuned to every person. We miss things; we have our own blind spots and strategies of disconnection; and we blunder. If so, as in all such instances, what matters is always what we do *next*, how we attempt to repair the situation or, as we would say, how we try to move the relationship from disconnection to new connection. Usually the way the therapist can attempt this movement is to be even more open and authentic about her own behavior and intent. The worst thing she can do is to pull away from connection, as Irene has described in an earlier paper on therapeutic impasses (Stiver, 1992).

CONCLUSION

Creative moments are important in therapy. But I want to emphasize that they are important as empowering acts in relation to the total society. While personal, they may lead people also to more understanding of a cultural system that restricts all of us–but in different ways for different groups of people. Just as this system restricts us, it prevents us from readily finding the ways to take action. That is, I believe that a cultural system built on the restriction of people by creating categories such as race, gender, class, and the like has thereby created a whole way of thinking and acting, in general, that inevitably leads to serious disconnection. This way of being structures even our most immediate personal experience. People still try to find connections in whatever ways they can but we inevitably build disconnections, strategies that keep us vigilant and restricted.

As Maureen Walker has pointed out, to be restricted–caught in these strategies–keeps us from finding new creative thought and action (Walker, 2000). When we are limited by our anxieties, we do not easily find the thoughts and actions that will lead us to create change in our lives and in the larger world. We are not likely to see the possibility of "the new."

These tendencies are, as always, what dominant-subordinate cultures engender. They first create conditions of oppression that lead to disconnections. They, then, lead us to the kinds of attempts at self-protection that keep us from finding alternatives, from finding new paths.

Most important, these strategies are attempts by each of us to try to find *individual* solutions and protections. They, thus, render us more disconnected. They keep us out of the creative and potentially joyous paths of acting together. In doing this kind of relational-cultural work, I hope we are learning more about how to replace disconnections with connections. I hope we can continue to extend this learning to realms beyond therapy to find new and better ways to work toward a more mutually empowering world for all of us.

REFERENCES

Bergman, S. (1990). Men's psychological development: A relational perspective. *Work in Progress, No. 48.* Wellesley, MA: Stone Center Working Paper Series.

Hartling, L. M., Rosen, W., Walker, M., & Jordan, J. V. (2000). Shame and humiliation: From isolation to relational transformation. *Work in Progress, No. 88.* Wellesley, MA: Stone Center Working Paper Series.

Jordan, J. V. (1989). Relational development: Therapeutic implications of empathy and shame. *Work in Progress, No. 39.* Wellesley, MA: Stone Center Working Paper Series.

Jordan, J. V., Kaplan, A. G., Miller, J. B., Stiver, I., & Surrey, J. (1991). *Women's growth in connection.* New York: Guilford Press.

Miller, J. B. (1988). Connections, disconnections, and violations. *Work in Progress, No. 33.* Wellesley, MA: Stone Center Working Paper Series.

Miller, J. B., & Stiver, I. P. (1994). Movement in therapy: Honoring the strategies of disconnection. *Work in Progress, No. 65.* Wellesley, MA: Stone Center Working Paper Series.

Miller, J. B., & Stiver, I. P. (1996). Relational images and their meanings. *Work in Progress, No. 74.* Wellesley, MA: Stone Center Working Paper Series.

Miller, J. B., & Stiver, I. P. (1997). *The healing connection.* Boston: Beacon Press.

Miller, J. B., Jordan, J. V., Stiver, I., Walker, M., Surrey, J., & Eldridge, N. (1999). Therapists' authenticity. *Work in Progress, No. 82.* Wellesley, MA: Stone Center Working Paper Series.

Stiver, I. P. (1992). A relational approach to therapeutic impasses. *Work in Progress, No. 58.* Wellesley, MA: Stone Center Working Paper Series.

Walker, M. (2000). Personal Communication.

What Changes in Therapy? Who Changes?

Natalie S. Eldridge
Janet L. Surrey
Wendy P. Rosen
Jean Baker Miller

SUMMARY. A central component of therapeutic change involves facilitating the capacity to move and be moved by the other. Another way of saying this might be that change entails experiencing a greater freedom of relational movement. The question of who and what actually changes in the process of therapy is the focus of the three vignettes that follow. They highlight, among other things, the recognition and acknowledgment of mutuality as an essential force within the relational matrix and the ever-changing landscape that this creates. Each of these examples of a change process bears, as well, a particular stamp of its own, and thus speaks to the unique personality of every therapeutic dyad.

Natalie S. Eldridge, PhD, is on the faculty of the Jean Baker Miller Training Institute, and a practicing psychologist.
Janet L. Surrey, PhD, is Founding Scholar and Faculty, JBMTI, and Attending Psychologist McLean Hospital/Harvard Medical School.
Wendy P. Rosen, PhD, is Attending Supervisor at McLean Hospital, and is in private practice in psychotherapy and supervision in Cambridge, MA.
Jean Baker Miller, MD (1927-2006), was Founding Scholar and Director of the Jean Baker Miller Training Institute at the Stone Center, Wellesley College; Clinical Professor of Psychiatry at Boston University School of Medicine; author of *Toward a New Psychology of Women*; and co-author of *The Healing Connection: How Women Form Relationships in Therapy and in Life*, and *Women's Growth in Connection*.

INTRODUCTION

By Jean Baker Miller, MD

The following vignettes offer clinical illustrations to suggest answers to the questions: What changes in therapy? Who changes? They formed part of a panel at the Learning from Women Conference sponsored by the Jean Baker Miller Training Institute and the Cambridge Hospital/Harvard Medical School Department of Continuing Medical Education in April, 2002. I introduced this panel by discussing some basic notions about the process of change and the obstacles to it on both the personal and societal levels.

Change is the essence of life. While it is most obvious in children, change is a necessity at all ages. It will happen inevitably. If we are ready to greet it, we can move to growth and joy; if not, we may encounter pain and trouble. Change toward growth creates pleasure; we feel most alive and zestful when we are moving in this expanding activity.

Growthful change usually occurs in interaction with others. People do not grow alone. According to Relational-Cultural Theory (RCT), change requires the ability to take in new experience occurring in these interactions and to construct new *relational images* (RIs). We have defined RIs as those inner constructions that we each create, often without awareness, out of our experience in relationships (Miller & Stiver, 1997). Beginning early in life we elaborate and complicate our RIs repeatedly. These images define what we expect will happen in relationships and also the meaning of this experience for our total selves, e.g., if we have had relationships that make us feel valuable, we carry over this meaning to make us feel worthy and confident in most realms of life such as school, work, and the like.

We probably compare new experience to the RIs we've created to date. If our RIs are relatively flexible as well as rich and nuanced, we then modify them. If they have been reinforced restrictively and repeatedly–and with strong emotional threat or harm, especially with psychological isolation–we may build more rigid RIs. These will be much harder to change.

Among other concepts about change in RCT are the *central relational paradox* (CRP) and *strategies of disconnection* (SDs; Miller & Stiver, 1997). The CRP states that people yearn to participate in connections with others but to the extent that their relationships have been unresponsive and/or hurtful, they will keep important parts of themselves out of connection–those parts that they believe are impossible to bring into relationship. SDs represent the many, varied ways we all develop to keep out of connection. The vignettes described in this article illustrate these concepts and others.

To consider influences on change, we have to look at the societal context. Patricia Hill Collins (2000), an African American sociologist, has written of *controlling images* (CIs) imposed on African American women, which Maureen Walker discussed in a recent paper (Walker & Miller, 2000). I believe this concept provides a valuable link between the social and psychological levels and can be extended to propose that we all live under CIs imposed by the dominant culture. However, CIs are different for each group in society. As we know, social groups are stratified, i.e., white upper-class men, white upper-class women, white middle-class men, and so on. CIs define for each group what is acceptable and what is not, what people can and cannot do. They exert a powerful impact on how we construct relationships, thus they heavily determine the RIs we create.

According to RCT, the most frightening human experience is psychological isolation. If severe, a person usually feels, along with isolation, a sense that she is the person at fault; she cannot be heard or understood; and she is powerless to change the situation. This is the meaning of "condemned isolation" (Miller, 1989). And this is a basic reason that change is so hard. While we may have many accompanying feelings, at bottom we fear that we will be rendered isolated and powerless. We fear altering our CIs, RIs, and SDs–those constructions that we believe we desperately need, that we think protect us from isolation. I believe this threat operates on our attempts to make change on both the societal and the individual psychological level.

The following vignettes sample some of the many aspects of change in therapy. While RCT offers many guides to therapeutic change, its central tenet is that each therapy will be unique as it evolves out of the particular relationship between patient and therapist. Thus, these illustrations do not provide concrete advice on specific topics. For example, with the person discussed here, Natalie Eldridge discovered that more "active listening" rather than verbal interventions led to more mutual connection. With another person, the opposite may be true. In the third example, Wendy Rosen is responding to a unique situation and would not necessarily be involved in gift giving with another person. As always, the most important feature was the growth of authenticity in connection that emerged out of the interchange around the gift.

All of these illustrations seek to counter the myth that the therapist is not affected by the therapeutic relationship. She certainly is, but *the purpose of therapy is to help the patient*. The therapist has the responsibility to act so that the relationship moves in a direction that is growth-fostering for the patient. In doing so and in trying to meet the patient at the point of her or his needs, the therapist may grow too.

VIGNETTE ONE: "MARY"

By Natalie S. Eldridge, PhD

Mary entered therapy in her early 30s to deal primarily with the task of coming out as a lesbian to her parents in the Midwest. She had moved to Boston about six months before in order to live with her current partner, Susan, with whom she had maintained a long-distance relationship for years. She described her history since graduating high school as one of distancing herself from her small-town roots and developing an urban lifestyle very foreign to her parents' experiences. While in a previous therapy in another city, she had come out to herself as a lesbian, but she kept this aspect of herself compartmentalized and hidden from her family. She did share her friendships and her work successes easily with them. This process of compartmentalizing actively reinforced her relational image that she maintained connection with others by not causing trouble and by being the adored little girl who is "bright, good, and nice." However, coming out to her parents had moved to the front burner for Mary in response to her deep commitment in her current relationship and her desire to share her happiness and success in love with her family. Her significant anxiety about the possible consequences of coming out to her family reflected the other dimension of her relational image: that bringing conflict or discomfort into relationship would leave her disconnected and isolated. This caused her a great deal of suffering and left her feeling paralyzed and frustrated in her desire to share her joy with them.

As our relationship developed, I came to understand the power that certain controlling images about being a lesbian had on her interactions with others. Her anxiety about the way she would be perceived by others, as "less than, sick, perverted, evil," was so painful to her sense of integrity, inherent goodness, and her deep religious and spiritual nature that she developed a strategy of disconnection (Miller & Stiver, 1997) with others to manage this anxiety. Her dominant relational image, influenced by these controlling images, might be described as: "If people see who I really am, as a lesbian and a sexual being, I will be punished, banished, discounted, and totally vulnerable." This image was so pervasive that I found it extending to her expectations about me, another lesbian whom she had carefully selected to be her therapist after interviewing at least three other lesbian-identified therapists.

In our relationship, a dominant strategy of disconnection emerged in which Mary managed her fear about being seen and judged by me by moving into passionate monologues about how unfair and unjust the laws and attitudes are toward lesbians and gay men, particularly regarding tolerance for love relationships. Whenever the topic of informing her family of the wonderful partnership she had with Susan would come up, her anxiety would skyrocket and she would share detailed stories of how she imagined anonymous others would view her if they knew about her sexuality. I came to see that her anxiety, which I submitted to the insurance company as a "diagnosis," was a by-product of her effort to counter or challenge her own strategy of disconnection. It functioned to keep parts of her hidden from those she feared would view her in a negative light at best and banish her at worst. This is the central relational paradox at work (Miller & Stiver, 1997). Mary was in therapy attempting to connect with me in preparation to share more fully with her family. Yet the very intention of doing so raised her anxiety and activated her strategies of disconnection so that she appeared to be working against her goals in the therapy *and* in interactions with family members.

I would like to say that I came to conceptually understand my work with Mary in the first months of therapy. However, Mary's strategies of disconnection were initially met with my own as I tried to negotiate the therapy relationship myself. As she launched into descriptive and eloquent monologues on her perception of homophobia and how "straight people think," I began to perceive our dynamic as a power-play in which Mary was casting me as the uninformed, if benign, therapist that she needed to educate. I developed my own image of this relational dynamic as Mary standing on a soapbox with me being an uncomfortable and silenced audience.

My resistance to this image and dynamic with Mary was reinforced by the controlling images I have internalized from my training that suggest the therapist needs to be in charge, at least half the time, and that story-telling is rarely useful in the therapy hour and needs to be redirected. I did not want to disconnect from Mary, but rather move toward a more authentic connection with her. So I was doing things like subtly redirecting the discussion as a way to stay engaged by reminding Mary of issues she wanted to work on. Unfortunately, these efforts would usually backfire, increasing her anxiety and serving to further rigidify her strategy of disconnection. Consequently, whenever the therapy hour seemed to be reduced to an intellectual discourse on discrimination, I was often left with my own feelings of shame.

Eventually, I began to recognize that my efforts to reinsert myself verbally to create a more mutual interaction with Mary were instead increasing her anxiety and her need to disconnect from mutual engagement with me. In fact, my interventions were a power play on my part, trying to regain a sense of control of the therapy process. I found I was trying to repair my own image of myself as a competent therapist. These attempts to reinsert myself into the dialogue were really "power-over" dynamics, reminding Mary of the difficulties that brought her into therapy and subtly suggesting she shouldn't be talking about what she was talking about. I was trying to get her to fit into my way of moving toward mutuality, but my way wasn't working. We needed to find a new pathway toward mutuality together.

At this point, I began to ask myself how I might try to repair the relationship. I began to recognize my own trigger of feeling silenced, represented in the relational image of Mary up on a soapbox while I am stuck in a silenced position. This was not a shared image, nor her image, but my image. As this became clearer, I worked to let go of this image of our dynamic. Instead of viewing myself as "being lectured to and silenced," I began to "revision" myself as a curious observer. This allowed me to grow more silent in the therapy, not inactive, but still and more fully present, and I began to resist less. As I sat with my curiosity about our relationship, I felt my deepening trust of Mary and my respect for her capacity to know what she needed. She had been showing me what she didn't need me to do, and I hadn't yet learned enough about how to move with her.

As I sat, an image emerged of myself as the cocounsel in a trial with Mary, the lead attorney–on the same team with her and there for support and to "hold the faith." Metaphorically speaking, I took myself out of the jury box to sit beside Mary as an ally as she delivered her perspective. This allowed me to engage without interfering or redirecting, thus responding in a new way. My own anxiety was calmed in the face of Mary's as I began to listen differently. I view this as an illustration of one way to shift power to move toward the potential for greater mutuality. This particular movement involved a de-escalation of my own strategies of disconnection. I was working to repair the relationship rather than repair my own image of how it "should be" (Miller, 2002).

Mary feels isolated; her acute awareness and fear of rejection leaves her feeling alone, and by fighting for understanding, she is also resisting her isolation. This, again, is her central relational paradox: she deeply desires and needs connection, acceptance, and celebration; yet, she is so fearful of potentially hurtful encounters with those important to her that she leaves large parts of who she is out of connection. Mary's old relational images were threatened and challenged by the therapy relationship; the idea of joining with a significant other person while making changes in herself violated her strategies of disconnection, which historically involved compartmentalizing her experience and rendering certain intimate conversations "off-limits."

As I began to understand the function of these strategies, I recognized that being a responsive listener to Mary involved being someone who is not shut down by her anxiety, nor needing to interrupt it, nor becoming swept up in it myself–that a *still presence* is essential to being with Mary in her experience to help her feel heard and understood. With this, my initial, anxious impatience with these interactions, where I felt "preached to," gave way to a deep compassion for Mary, and I realized how difficult it was for her to feel safe. Our new dynamic allowed me to be invited in, rather than trying to "redirect" the energy of her strategy of disconnection. My work as the therapist required becoming more responsive to her movement, noticing and letting go of my own impulse to react, and refocusing on simply listening and staying present. I was holding the faith in Mary and in the relational process while I was holding Mary's anxiety without giving it more power. In the process, I became more attuned to Mary's subtle shifts to protect her sense of safety. Our relationship now had more space for movement toward mutuality in her way and at her pace. This gave me room to be ready to move with her when she was ready to move.

In one session, a couple years into therapy, we began to discuss how Mary's family members might react or respond to her coming out to them. (She was no longer talking off the point.) She was elaborating on the communication system in her family. In her childhood, she said they lived in a large farmhouse in which seven siblings had their own rooms, but *were never allowed to close their doors*. I had a deep gut response to this image, a sudden and poignant grasping of her sense of vulnerability and the lack of safety she experienced as result of never being able to retreat behind a closed door. My internal response was a mixture of my own strong valuation of and need for privacy and my concern about how intrusive this family rule felt to me combined. This triggered a metaphorical light bulb going off in our relationship that eventually helped us both understand that Mary's anxiety was a way to prevent others from seeing what she wasn't prepared to reveal. She had developed strategies that actually functioned as doors that could provide a sense of privacy, allowing only invited intimacy to enter. This was a moment of a felt sense of "we"–discovering together the impact of the open door policy in her childhood. In this moment she felt me feeling with her, as we moved together into greater understanding. I think of a moment like this as experienced evidence of the movement toward mutuality in the relationship.

Several years into our work, Mary was able to come out to her family. Together we reviewed many changes and shifts in her life that contributed to her readiness to take this step, that is, her readiness to make relational shifts. One significant shift occurred in response to the unexpected illness and death of her father, with whom she felt the greatest fear of loss in coming out. She was able to negotiate his last months with a presence and intimacy that they had rarely experienced in their relationship and made her peace with him without a formal disclosure about her sexuality.

Another significant relational shift was the deepening of trust and commitment in her relationship with Susan. Mary moved from a rather fixed and feared relational image of herself as "single" and unloved–an image she believed her family would see as her fate as a lesbian and an image she had internalized despite the reality of her relationship with Susan–to an increasingly internalized image of herself within a committed and solid relationship. This drastically changed her sense of power and status vis-à-vis her family–though it didn't change her family's religious views of gay lifestyles or non-heterosexual marriages.

A third shift occurred through our relational work together. Rather than viewing her anxiety and obsessive worry as a pathological process, Mary began to see her experience as a unique process that often provided her with a reasonable and effective method for reaching her goals. This became a new relational image of her relationship with herself that allowed her to find ways to intervene to reduce the *unnecessary* anxiety while celebrating the way she "does her worrying upfront" in a preventive manner. As a result, she became empowered enough in the relational contexts she encountered to feel less vulnerable to the potential judgment and biases of family and culture. This cognitive, or visionary, shift came about through movement toward mutuality in our relationship and allowed her greater flexibility in her relational images. She gained courage in connection, which provided her with the conditions for growthful change.

What Changed for Mary?

Mary and I discussed the question of how change happens in therapy. She responded with a written list of some of the ways she experienced change in our work together. I will share this list verbatim as a way to bring her voice more directly into this presentation. I invite you to listen for the voices of some of your clients in Mary's words.

According to Mary, here are some of the ways in which change happened in therapy:

1. I felt I was truly seen and heard for who I am. This, in and of itself, was enormously healing.
2. I always sensed your "hopefulness," Natalie–an optimism about me on your part when I didn't see a path to resolution or a solution or a change ever coming myself.
3. Natalie–you are a skilled listener. You really heard me and related aspects of what I told you about myself to a larger picture of me and my world. Your listening and insight showed me you were really engaged in my situation. That helped me trust the safety of the relationship and the sense that I was not being judged.
4. You were able to identify patterns for me that I was unable to see myself. You showed real insight into me and my ways of doing things.
5. Since you could understand what I was feeling or doing, I came to believe that those actions and choices couldn't be entirely random or senseless, but instead, part of a somewhat predictable course of action. Once we could predict the course of action, or at least recognize where we were along the well-traveled route, two things happened for me: I calmed down–my anxiety subsided although the situations hadn't significantly changed, and we could identify ways to change the pattern.
6. A big part of change happening for me was that I believed it would. I had some measure of "proof" that change could happen from my previous therapy and for some reason, I simply believed that this would work.

7. Natalie–I always felt liked and appreciated. I always felt like our therapy sessions were a special project we'd taken on together and I never felt like anything but your top priority.
8. I learned some gentleness from you–patience with myself (which became patience with others) and I learned to give credit where credit is due. When I made progress in my life, you helped me learn to acknowledge it.
9. I feel you held my fears and sorrows and joys and triumphs very tenderly and respectfully, and you truly rejoiced with me when I grew and good things happened for me. I'll always be grateful for the fruit of our work–what we discovered together. Thank you.

Conclusions

In summary, I want to acknowledge Mary for her patience and persistence in our relationship, which allowed me to become a better therapist. I also want to acknowledge Mary for engaging in a relational process that allowed us both to grow, though in different ways. One of the things that changed for me in the therapy relationship was gaining a clearer picture of my own reactive triggers around feeling silenced or verbally "left out" of connection. Other therapy relationships had not been so dynamically stuck around this sense of disconnection. Other clients either were less persistent in lecturing me or responded to my efforts to bring myself into the conversation with increased engagement, rather than greater disconnection. So I was able to expand my own understanding of myself in this relationship and, thus, I was able to move from a stance of resistance (being her audience) to one of attunement and helpful engagement. This experience has since been salient in my other relationships, both therapeutic and personal, giving me greater flexibility in my responses and expanding the relational possibilities.

I appreciate Mary's faith in the therapy process, which she brought into our work from a past therapy relationship. I am thankful for my numerous past therapeutic relationships, in which I was either the therapist or the client, that allowed me to strengthen my faith in relational change. It was the expansive growth in these previous relationships that Mary experienced as my "optimism," my sense of "hopefulness" in our work together. I think of this optimism as the capacity *to hold the faith in a relationship* (Stiver, 1992). Each of us draws from our experiences in relational contexts, both the expansive and the restrictive, to bring forth the unique chemistry in each new connection. What changes in therapy?

Who changes? I believe that in the kind of mutually empathic connection described by Relational-Cultural Theory, the therapist and the client are both changed in an expansive and zestful way, and that this change is carried by both therapist and client to others far beyond the therapy room.

VIGNETTE TWO: "HELEN"

By Janet L. Surrey, PhD

Natalie has described the extraordinary opportunities for change, growth, and expansion within the therapy relationship–for both client and therapist. We all speak of the risks and challenges in this work, but tend to emphasize the overall arc of the healing relationship as a mutually expanding, redeeming, and creative movement. We need also to highlight the complexities and difficulties. I want to take the risk today of talking about a challenging, ongoing, long-term, therapy relationship with a client I'll call "Helen."

In my 25 years as a clinician, I have experienced a small number of relationships that stand out as exceptionally difficult, that have challenged me to the core. These have involved a high intensity of emotional connection, as well as extreme doubt and disconnection for the client and, simultaneously, for me. The client comes to experience therapy and the relationship itself as both very healing and empowering and for significant periods, very hurtful and harmful. For these clients, therapy evokes intense longings for connection that do not feel truly met, gratified, or "held" sufficiently in the relationship. The intensity of the pain and deprivation surrounding the longings resonate with the client's early relational experience and comes to feel unbearable, humiliating, and even re-wounding. At times, the intensity of the therapy feels as if it *is* the problem; that is, it is interfering with the rest of the client's life.

The first challenge for me becomes my own capacity to stay with, bear witness to, and validate the client's pain without resorting to strategies of disconnection around pathologizing the client ("she's a real borderline") or myself ("I'm so inadequate . . . I should be doing other work"), devaluing therapy as a process, or fantasizing about standing in front of a malpractice jury defending myself. Without these strategies, I am left to remain "present" and take a long hard look at the potentially harmful aspects of therapy (for both the client and myself).

I have always been able to call on Irene Stiver for help in these situations. It is particularly painful to feel her absence today–though clearly her presence is still so powerful. As a supervisor and consultant, she made it easy for us to ask for help when we were having difficulties.

She helped normalize and detoxify the shame around impasses and suggested structural changes such as adding a co-therapist when necessary or even sometimes ending a therapy relationship with a transfer to another therapist. She was so full of energy, curiosity, and extraordinary faith in this process, which always helped me to stay with it, see openings for new movement, and sense subtle changes. She was always willing to help us and our clients acknowledge frustration, resentment, doubt, and despair that can emerge in such relationships, and are perhaps a necessary part of the work. Irene's relational presence and faith are still with me in the relationship I will talk about today, as it was the last one I shared with her.

My relationship with Helen began six years ago when she was 39. At the time, she was referred by a colleague who had met her at a workshop for women over 40 considering first time motherhood. Helen had become aware of her deep fears–even terror–of becoming a mother. Having a doctoral degree in experimental psychology, she worked as a very successful scientist and manager in a large corporate setting. She described herself as very competent and well-organized, a real "doer." She had little tolerance for people who couldn't take action to solve problems.

Helen had met her husband in graduate school, and they had been married for 11 years. She described the relationship as very compatible and comfortable. They shared professional interests, a deep love of nature and sports, spent time together hiking and traveling, and took care of their two well-loved golden retrievers. Helen had few women friends. She recognized that she stayed away from her feelings and withdrew from relationships that became too close, where she felt too hopeful, vulnerable, or mistrustful. As she began to trust me and to talk about her family, particularly her mother, the intensity of our relationship grew, and this seemed appropriate and touching.

Helen was emotionally removed from and critical of her parents– though still in ongoing contact with them. As the second daughter, she felt she had always been a great disappointment to her mother who was hoping for a son. Her two younger brothers were born five and seven years later. She described herself as profoundly alienated and critical of her mother whom she felt was frightening, disorganized, and far away– "we live in different worlds." From birth, she felt that her mother was intensely bonded with Helen's older sister, whom Helen felt had been psychologically abusive and threatening to her as a child. There was "no room" for her in this sister-mother dyad, and Helen felt that they both viewed her as unfeeling, critical, and rejecting. This relational image led her to doubt herself and to worry about being a "poison person," who could be hateful, rejecting, and destructive of relationships.

From infancy, she felt more bonded and identified with her father, who was her "great hope," but the relationship was more fantasy than reality. Helen's father turned out to be an active alcoholic who created a great scandal for the family in a very public affair when Helen was an adolescent. He disappointed her deeply, and their relationship virtually died at that time. Helen built her life around her capacity to perform at school, to take care of the younger boys, and then to get out of the family and become as different as possible from both her parents.

In our third year of therapy, just as she made the decision to try to become pregnant, Helen's husband was diagnosed with leukemia–a very slow-growing but ultimately life threatening form–and one of their dogs was killed in a freak accident. These events brought plans for a family to a halt and initiated a profound personal, relational, and spiritual crisis. Through this terrible time and its aftermath she began to feel very dependent on me (wanting much extra time and many out of session phone calls), painfully vulnerable, and often enraged. Helen's pain and grief felt unbearable to her at times and evoked her overwhelming longings to be held, comforted, and "mothered" by me.

Helen felt very pained by these longings, shamed by their intensity, and deeply disappointed with my failures to respond in the way she had desired. At times she sensed that I felt overwhelmed and overburdened by her; this would trigger a major disconnection that could last a few minutes, a few weeks, or a few months. Watching and gauging her impact on me, she was sensitive and vigilant to every nuance in my attentiveness or emotional availability.

My Journey with Helen

I had been called to accompany Helen through an intensity of suffering and despair, disconnection, and hopelessness that could feel unbearable to me too. At times, I have felt resentful about the energy and care I had given to this relationship. The depth of her anger and her strategies to deal with her own feelings of powerlessness evoked my strategies of disconnection–strategies to avoid, withdraw, or even subtly retaliate.

Hardest for me were the times when she needed to tell me in great detail how hurt she has been by me (and I recognized that she needed to test me with this over and over to see that I wouldn't turn it back on her the way her mother did). My own strategy of disconnection in response to this was to become frustrated and irritated, and then to move into a shame reaction, a kind of freeze or disengagement meant to avoid further harm and to assess the situation. She sensed this, felt me "go away" psychologically, and then she felt abandoned. We were both contending with controlling cultural images of women (especially mothers) who are *never* supposed to hurt or harm others and the controlling images of therapists who are always supposed to be clear, self-aware, in control, always having faith in therapy and who are especially *not harmful*. I knew these images were oppressive and unreal but still I wrestled with them, particularly in the hardest times when struggling with such complexities and contradictions.

I had to acknowledge to her that there *are* structural limitations in therapy, just as there are structural supports. The dyadic structure does not always work in positive ways. Particularly, holding pain like this takes "a whole village," or a whole family and community, which simply did not exist, for her. And there were inequalities and power differentials between us. She was in a more vulnerable position. I could go home to members of my family, who are my priority. I didn't need her in the same way she needed me. She *was* expected to share all her feelings and I was not. I had real limits on my availability for out of session contact. These constraints were not about her unreasonable neediness, but are the real limits, inequalities, and asymmetries built into the structure of therapy. Further, my limits as a person and a therapist are very observable and have real impact.

In every therapy, there is a shared grieving process for what cannot or does not change, occurring simultaneously with the movements of real growth and expansion. This relationship demands a great deal from both of us in this shared task of grieving together and mutual acceptance of limits. No matter how much personal and clinical work I have done, I often feel I am struggling to participate moment to moment with Helen in this delicate and sometimes dangerous dance of mutual movement.

In Relational-Cultural Theory we say that as the relationship changes, the people change. What do we mean when we say the relationship has changed? For this, I use the language of "We." Each of us and the relationship, the We, have expanded and contracted through this mutual movement. Helen has been pushed to let go of old protective strategies of disconnection, as have I. She has touched her depths and has survived, so far. We have both hurt and cared for each other. There have been some extraordinary and redeeming moments of profound connection, compassion, insight, forgiveness, and love. There have been times of major disconnection and steps toward reconnection that have felt excruciatingly painful and not always clearly growth-fostering.

We have touched bottom together. We have grown in our ability to look at and talk about the disconnects together, even as they occur, without having to re-enact them all the way. This reflects growth in relational awareness–as we "draw the map of the relationship" together–mapping out the places where the We is strong and resilient and places where the We feels fragile or severed. We may never be able to avoid these places, but can learn to manage them with somewhat greater awareness and care, beginning to hold the We together through the disconnects. The relationship grows through shared vulnerability and humility towards deeper levels of compassion for each other and for the relationship.

Neither of us can do it alone. We can learn better to do it together. We can learn to let go of obstacles together and reenter these painful places where we each feel like failures and to build on the moments of connection, trust, and mutual respect. Through this, the relationship grows in empowerment and resilience–generating emotional and spiritual resources to draw on as we work through the places of isolation and darkness, holding the faith that something new can grow here. In some ways, the growth in the We is not under either of our control. There is always a mystery, a grace in the movement.

For both of us, this shift to the We was a place of refuge, out of the terrible isolation of shame and blame, out of power and control battles subtle and obvious. Helen's journey from "You," to "I," to "We" has been more visible to me lately. From "You are hurting me," to "I am in terrible pain," to the recent question that truly touched and inspired me: "Can't we find a way to do this better?"

I think Jean Baker Miller's use of Patricia Hill Collins (2000) image of clinical work as "visionary pragmatism" is very apt. It is truly a challenge to hold the vision and faith in the possibility of relational growth while staying open to explore the places of real doubt, loss of hope, and the inevitable grief that lies in the disparity between the vision and the reality.

VIGNETTE THREE: "MAURA"

By Wendy P. Rosen, PhD

At its best, meeting in mutual vulnerability in the therapy relationship can level the playing field and sow the seeds of relational change and growth. It is in just such a meeting place that I choose to speak of my relationship with Maura. Maura is a savvy business person who comes from a working-class, Irish Catholic background with a history of extreme poverty and survival sensibility on both sides of her family. I, on the other hand, am a "feeling doctor" coming from a middle-class, Eastern European Jewish background with a history of flight from persecution on both sides of my family and the attendant sense of fear, mistrust, and quiet self-deprecation that this engenders. Both of us are lesbians in an oppressively homophobic culture, which further exacerbates this image of the precarious nature of safe, loving, and enduring relationships.

Maura came in one day and handed me a copy of a quote that she has pinned up in her office. It described the lives of the gazelle and the lion; running to stay alive.

In return, I recited for Maura a poem by Charles Simic that has inspired me for years: It speaks to a sense of not belonging; of seeking roots.

The quotes we shared represent, among other things, something about our own core relational images. Furthermore, they speak to a more historical context of controlling images suggested by the dominant culture about the collective fates of both the Irish and the Jewish immigrant in this country. While these appear to be very different relational images for Maura and me, hers suggesting relational fight or flight in the competition for survival and mine speaking to a kind of Diaspora-like sense of rootlessness, both speak to the risk or instability we were bred to fear on some visceral level about relationships.

One difference between Maura and me, however, has to do with our particular strategies of disconnection. Maura's framework is one of power over, while mine is one of inefficacy and alienation. It's not that either one of us is a stranger to the other's protective strategies. Rather, it is that each of us has learned to lead with a particular relational stance in the face of uncertainty due in part to the kinds of early connections, disconnections, cultural contexts, and resultant relational images we have known. What we share in common without question, however, is the sense that meeting in vulnerability is a risky and unreliable endeavor. A fundamental struggle for each of us is whether or not meeting in vulnerability with another can truly be a growth-promoting relational experience, that is, one of positive and enduring change. It is, after all, one of the great paradoxes of life, that to change and grow, we must be open and vulnerable to one another, the very context in which our relational injuries have occurred.

Empathic meetings require a certain mutual permeability, an openness to influence, the allowance for a shared state of vulnerability. One way that Maura deals with her mostly unspoken emotional hunger is through her tremendous generosity. On the one hand, it is a genuine, essential, core part of her. It is also true that this same generosity can sometimes serve to keep her from knowing the true emotional reciprocity of a loving relationship. The net result is that she doesn't get to see if a relationship can grow and survive in response to something other than such giving, or whether or not she has something of emotional value to offer, or whether she might be freely given to simply for who she is.

Maura knows less about loving a person into survival and growth than about providing for someone's survival and growth. Maura has given me gifts that have been thoughtful and generous. I've felt both touched and uncomfortable. I've shared with her my appreciation, but also, my fear that she will feel that she has to give me presents in order for me to value her and our relationship. She counters my cautious protests with statements of acknowledgment that I "always go the extra mile" with her whenever she needs it, extending the hour, talking on the phone or reaching out when I know she cannot. What she doesn't get to feel from me, however, is that she, in fact, touches me powerfully.

One way that I deal with my nagging sense of inadequacy about the worth of what I have to give is through minimizing both my acts of generosity in life and their value. It is my attempt to protect myself by preempting others in what I fear will be their devaluation of my emotional investment. At the same time, it doesn't allow for any felt sense of efficacy on my part in the way of empathic connections or the feeling of power in the gift of my own emotional responsiveness. In other words, our own anxious efforts at feeling worthwhile in relationships entail strategies of self-protection and disengagement. Maura, on some level, feels unworthy of being given to emotionally, and I struggle with feeling that there is little worth to what I have to give. While I try to challenge this default setting of mine, I'm not always successful.

At Christmas this past year, I gave Maura a present to give to her niece, Cara, whom she is raising on her own. Cara's mother, Maura's younger sister, has a significant substance abuse problem and cannot safely care for her daughter. I'd given Maura a couple of small gifts in the past for no special reason, except that they made me think of her. Whenever I did this, Maura seemed a bit nonchalant in her response, thanking me but then quickly moving on to other things. I was struck by what seemed like discomfort of some sort, although I never openly addressed the feeling. When I gave the Christmas present to her, I found myself thoroughly downplaying it, saying it was just a "little thing" for her niece, "no big deal," "just a little something." In point of fact, it was not an elaborate gift in the concrete sense, but it was meaningful nonetheless. Maura's response was exactly the same as in the past, and we seamlessly moved on. This time, however, the giving came from a different place in me, that is, one of being moved by what I experienced as something powerfully touching for me about Maura. It had to do with Maura's relationship with her niece and my sense of how deeply loving, devoted, and self-sacrificing she has been in the service of giving her niece a chance at a good life. Maura's loving generosity moved me deeply.

At our next session, I found myself a little irrationally hurt that I hadn't heard from Maura about her niece's response to the gift. She had barely sat down in her chair, when I impulsively asked her about it. She shifted uncomfortably and said to me, "Well, we opened it, and what I want to know is whether somebody gave that to you, and you didn't want it, so you handed it down to us." I recall feeling stunned, wounded, ashamed, and defensive. She said that she and Cara had hung up the gift, and then we moved on and talked about absolutely nothing that I can remember. At that point, I had become emotionally disengaged and remained there for the rest of the hour, while unconvincingly trying to seem as if I were present. At the end of that day, I felt deeply upset about Maura's response. I decided initially that I was being far too sensitive and vulnerable and that I needed to go off on my own, somehow get my reaction under control, and understand it better. Realizing what a dead end that was going to be, I told a very close friend and colleague about the interaction. She helped me to move back into the relationship with Maura by recognizing something of the mutually shared, relational elements to this event, that is, that something was touched off between us which stemmed from some more hidden place of mutual vulnerability.

I talked to Maura at our next appointment about what had occurred. I told her that her response had left me feeling hurt, but that I did not think that my feelings were entirely a reaction to her words. I said that I had spoken with a colleague/friend of mine about it in order to try and make sense of the interaction. Most important was the fact that I had moved out of connection with her, and I wanted to make my way back into our relationship. After exclaiming, "God, you're so sensitive!" to which I offered no argument, we proceeded to begin the slow and careful work of peeling away the layers of each of our responses.

Maura was right. I am sensitive, and it sometimes dovetails with an early relational image of mine that defined emotional sensitivity as too vulnerable a place in which to be, that is, as a personal liability, subject to being exploited, shamed, and wounded. On the other hand, it is also a trait that helps me to be a caring and thoughtful therapist. I suggested to Maura that sensitivity can render one vulnerable to hurt, but that it is also a good thing in relationships, allowing for real contact.

Maura took that in and thought about it, coming back the next time with a list of responses she had to our interaction. These included:

1. I thought it was safe to talk. I didn't think about your feelings.
2. I never even had my coat off.
3. Yes, I'm a little slow at expressing that emotion (i.e., gratitude), but whose time clock do I need to be on?
4. You set me up by minimizing and devaluing gifts you give me.
5. You disconnected from me during our session, and it says on page 32 or something of that book you gave me (*The Healing Connection*) that that's not a good thing.
6. What hurts me the most is that you didn't talk to me first about your feelings, that you didn't trust me enough and had to go to someone else instead.

Her list of feeling observations was truly on the money and felt like her finest gift to date. I told her how much I appreciated what she'd given me and that her list was worthy of even deeper examination in order to understand something important about our relationship and relationships in general. This, of course, made her groan, muttering, "Can't we just move on to something else?"

I believe there are a few important points about this series of interactions that speak to the subject of power and change in therapy. First, it sheds light on the very complex reality of what two people bring to a relationship; that is, the many layers of personal relational images that come into contact with one another and at the point of intersection, carry the potential to create either healthy change or damaging acts of power abuse. Second, it speaks to the deeply vulnerable places around which our strategies of relational disconnection are organized and act to keep us apart from one another. Third, it underscores both the inevitability and opportunity of meeting in places of shared vulnerability as a catalyst for real change, both in the movement of the relationship, as well as in the individual relational images of each person in the relationship.

Places of vulnerability are not simply about old relational wounds, but rather about old wounds remaining open, even in the present. It is the willing reciprocity of sometimes painful openness, of shared movement toward real authenticity and an allowance to be modified by this experience that provides the opportunities for relational repair and expansion.

Maura and I are still very much in this process, but change is already occurring. We know that there are times when we will fail each other. It is our willing examination of these failures that deepens our perspectives on the rich complexity of feelings and old images that are brought to bear in the ongoing life of any relationship. I've been learning a lot about my vulnerable places and my strategies of disconnection in the face of them. In particular, I'm seeing the deep complexity for me of what generosity and giving of myself actually represent, and also, the maladaptive ways in which I try to preempt my most feared responses while paradoxically creating them. It has freed me to go further with Maura about my experience of her and to more freely give voice to my observations, treating them as valuable and meaningful gifts toward relational growth.

Maura, too, is changing. She is looking at her influence on important people in her life in a new way, allowing herself to pause long enough to feel their experiences, especially in response to her, and to bear them, moving further into real empathy and expanding her own inherent sense of value and worth. Our relationship has expanded to include loving admiration, caring, and mutual inspiration even in the face of disappointments, and it has been rendered stronger by the repairs we allow and create together.

REFERENCES

Collins, P. H. (2000). Black feminist thought (2nd ed.). New York: Routledge.
Miller, J. B. (1988). Connections, disconnection, and violations. Work in Progress, No. 33. Wellesley, MA: Stone Center Working Paper Series.
Miller, J. B. (2002). How change happens: Controlling images, mutuality, and power. Work in Progress, No. 96. Wellesley, MA: Stone Center Working Paper Series.
Miller, J. B., & Stiver, I. P. (1997). The healing connection. Boston: Beacon Press.
Simic, C. (1971). Dismantling the silience. New York: Brazziler.
Sparks, E. (1998). Against all odds: Resistance and resilience in African American welfare mothers. Work in Progress, No. 81. Wellesley, MA: Stone Center Working Paper Series.
Stiver, I. P. (1992). A relational approach to therapeutic impasses. Work in Progress, No. 58. Wellesley, MA: Stone Center Working Paper Series.
Walker, M., & Miller, J. B. (2000). Racial images and relational possibilities. Talking Paper, No. 2. Wellesley, MA: Stone Center Working Paper Series.

Strengthening Resilience in a Risky World: It's All About Relationships

Linda M. Hartling

SUMMARY. Building on Judith Jordan's earlier work on relational resilience, this paper challenges the commonly held view that resilience is a unique form of individual "toughness" endowed to a lucky few and suggests that resilience can be strengthened in all people through participation in growth-fostering relationships. The author reviews the research describing individual, internal characteristics associated with resilience and explores the relational aspects of these characteristics. A case example illustrates that efforts promoting relational development help people grow through and beyond experiences of hardship and adversity. In addition, the author proposes specific ways resilience can be strengthened through engagement in relationships that enhance one's intellectual development, sense of worth, sense of competence, sense of empowerment, and, most importantly, sense of connection.

Linda M. Hartling, PhD, is Associate Director of the Jean Baker Miller Training Institute; member of the Board of Directors of Human Dignity and Humiliation Studies; and co-editor of *The Complexity of Connection*.

INTRODUCTION

In 1992 when Judith Jordan wrote about relational resilience as a "life-giving empathic bridge," she offered a profound reframing of the source of human ability to overcome adversities, hardships, and trauma. She challenged us to move beyond a highly circumscribed focus on individual, internal traits to a broader and deeper examination of the relational dynamics that promote growth in the face of hardship. According to Jordan:

> we can no longer look only at factors within the individual which facilitate adjustment; we must examine the relational dynamics that encourage the capacity for connection. (p. 1)

> Few studies have delineated the complex factors involved in those relationships, which not only protect us from stress but also promote positive and creative growth. (p. 3)

Rather than perpetuating the common notion of resilience as some form of intrinsic toughness endowed to a few unique or heroic individuals, Jordan opened the way to understanding resilience as a human capacity that can be developed and strengthened in *all* people through relationships, specifically through growth-fostering relationships.

Today, Jordan's reconceptualization of resilience leads us to a profoundly valuable source of hope and courage as we face accumulating evidence that we are living in a riskier world (e.g., terrorist threats, global economic instability and injustice, civil unrest, extreme global climate changes, violent international conflict, widespread destruction of natural resources, corporate corruption, and world-wide epidemics, as well as intractable hunger and poverty). Just as more researchers are becoming more keenly aware of how trauma, hardships, and adversities can derail the lives of children and adults (Banks, 2000; Bremmer, 2002), more individuals, families, and communities are facing forms of threat that were once unthinkable. Today, growing numbers of people have palpable fears about a repeat of the 9/11 tragedy; random rampage shootings; possible nuclear/biological/chemical weapons attacks; suicide bombings around the world; outbreaks of intractable, incurable diseases; etc. Given these developments, people cannot afford to wager that they are blessed with superior fortitude (individual resilience). Rather, all of us can find ways to strengthen our resilience *now* by developing our capacity to build healthy connections with others, our families, and our communities, that is, by developing our relational resilience (Jordan, 1992).

Based on a review of the research, this article will explore the popular construction of resilience as an individual commodity and propose an alternate view: resilience as a relational activity. It will describe and examine the individual characteristics that are commonly associated with resilience and offer a relational understanding of these characteristics. Furthermore, it will be begin to identify specific ways to strengthen resilience through relationships. Although this discussion is framed within the context of therapy, readers are encouraged to extend their thinking beyond confines of clinical practice. Because, as this article proposes, in or out of therapy, *resilience is all about relationships.*

You are invited to begin this discussion with a brief activity to tap into your own experience of resilience. Please take a moment to respond to the following questions:

1. Reflect on a time when you felt someone contributed to your ability to be resilient after experiencing a loss, hardship, disappointment, or difficulty. What types of things did that person do that made the difference?
2. Reflect on a time when you felt like you contributed to someone else's ability to be resilient after experiencing a loss, hardship, disappointment, or difficulty. What types of things did you do that you think made the difference?

Please keep your reflection in mind as we continue our discussion by examining the research on resilience.

FROM INDIVIDUAL STRENGTHS TO STRENGTHENING RELATIONSHIPS

The literature primarily defines resilience in two different ways. First, resilience is described as the ability to achieve good outcomes in one's life after experiencing significant hardships or adversities, such as poverty, family discord, divorce, lack of access to educational opportunities, racism, etc. Within this definition, a "good outcome" for some individuals would be the absence of deviant and anti-social behavior. Another common definition suggests that resilience is the ability to recover from traumatic experiences, such as physical or sexual abuse, assault, severe neglect, and many other forms of trauma. These definitions tend to generate the notion of resilience as something located within the individual, some type of special individual competence or strength. From this perspective, the interest in individual characteristics and strengths moves to the foreground.

The tendency to focus on individual strengths in the study of resilience is reinforced by traditional Western-European theories of psychological development that have historically emphasized individual development and experience. Most of these theories hold the underlying assumption that the goal of healthy development is to separate from relationships in order to become an independent, self-sufficient, i.e., strong adult (Jordan, 1992; Cushman, 1995). Consequently, these theories of development tend to lead researchers and clinicians to spotlight the experience of the *self*, the individual, while relational experience is relegated to the background and is all too often ignored. Within a scientific tradition that places relational experience on the periphery, researchers become absorbed in efforts to identify and describe characteristics located within the individual. With regard to resilience, much research focuses on identifying "special strengths," such as intelligence, good-natured temperament, higher self-esteem, internal locus of control, mastery, etc. This approach to the study of resilience promotes the belief that the lucky few, *those endowed with these special strengths,* will succeed, will be resilient, and will become independent and self-sufficient despite encounters with significant obstacles. The rest of us may be out of luck. But something is missing from this picture. How do people develop the strengths associated with resilience? Certainly, these strengths are not entirely inherent. Certainly, these strengths are not developed in isolation.

The Relational-Cultural Theory (RCT) of psychological development offers a new foundation for understanding the research on resilience. RCT proposes that healthy development involves the formation and elaboration of growth-fostering relationships throughout one's life. RCT moves us beyond a myopic emphasis on individual development and individual strengths and encourages the study of *relational development* and *relational strengths*. RCT would propose that relationships are a primary source of one's ability to be resilient in the face of personal and social hardships or trauma. Furthermore, relationships are a primary source of experiences that strengthen the individual characteristics commonly associated with resilience. In many ways, process of effective psychotherapy is an example of how resilience is strengthened through relationship.

An RCT approach to understanding resilience includes understanding the complexities of how people establish, engage in, and sustain growth-fostering (or resilience-strengthening) relationships throughout their lives. In particular, RCT suggests that all relationships are constructed within, and are highly defined by, the social and cultural contexts in which they exist. A cultural context can facilitate or obstruct one's opportunities to participate in relationships necessary for strengthening one's ability to be resilient. For example, as Maureen Walker (2000) explains, cultural contexts in which stratification of difference is enforced by dominant-subordinate systems of power undermine opportunities to engage in growth-fostering relationships. Being a member of a subordinate or marginalized group increases the risk that one's relationships will be chronically or acutely disrupted by adversities, such as poverty, lack of educational opportunities, institutionalized discrimination, insufficient health care, etc. Furthermore (so-called) objective observers, such as researchers, are not immune to the influences of dominant-subordinate power arrangements in a society. Jean Baker Miller (1976) observed that, "... the close study of an oppressed group reveals that a dominant group inevitably describes the subordinate group falsely in terms derived from its own systems of thought" (p. xix). Thus, researchers may conduct studies that implicitly privilege the individual characteristics of dominant group as the norm or ideal, while missing other important factors. For instance, in a cultural context in which the dominant group values individual achievement and independence, relational factors may be disregarded or dismissed (Fletcher, 1999). The following example illustrates this point.

In the 1970s, Kobasa (1979; Kobasa & Puccetti, 1983) identified an individual, internal characteristic associated with resilience to stress called "hardiness." A "hardy" individual, according to Kobasa (1979), exhibits three characteristics:

1. Commitment: being able to easily commit to what one is doing
2. Control: a general belief that events are within one's control and
3. Challenge: perceiving change as a challenge rather than a threat.

The concept of hardiness was well received in academic and clinical communities, and over the years hardiness has been used as a standard of stress resilience applied across diverse populations of men, women, and children. Yet, today we are aware of the limitations of this initial research. Kobasa's work was based on the study of a narrowly defined group, specifically white male middle- to upper-level business executives. While the individual characteristics of commitment, control, and challenge (i.e., hardiness) appeared to be useful for describing stress resilience of the subjects in the initial research, unfortunately the conclusions derived from this research triggered "faulty generalizations" imposed on other populations (Minnich, 1990). The individual characteristic of hardiness may not be an accurate measure of the experience of women and others not represented in the study. Furthermore, today we are conscious of the social/cultural context in which this research was conducted. In the 1970s business executives were the beneficiaries of invisible systems of relational support comprised of secretaries, wives, mothers, and undervalued service providers (experts in providing relational support) who likely made it possible for these privileged professionals to be "hardy."

If the hardiness researchers had investigated a diverse population, they might have identified many other characteristics associated with stress resilience. For example, Elizabeth Sparks (1999) explored the resilience of African American mothers on welfare and described the relational practices these women used to survive tremendous hardships. These mothers engaged in connection, collaboration, and community action to overcome the destructive impact of poverty, racism, and social stigmatization. While traditional theories of development have led many researchers–although not all researchers–to emphasize the study of individual traits associated with resilience, RCT suggests that researchers can enlarge, deepen, and enrich their understanding of resilience by examining the relational-cultural factors that contribute to one's ability to be resilient. Taking an RCT perspective might ultimately lead to defining resilience as *the ability to connect, reconnect, and resist disconnection in response to hardships, adversities, trauma, and alienating social/cultural practices*. This definition opens the way to new possibilities for strengthening resilience in the lives of individuals, families, and communities. It moves us beyond hoping that people will have the "right stuff," that is, the individual strengths to be resilient in a risky world–to identifying practices that strengthen the relationships that foster resilience in our risky world.

RELATIONALLY RETHINKING INDIVIDUAL RESILIENCE

Taking a relational-cultural view of resilience offers us the opportunity to reexamine and rethink the meaning of the existing research on resilience. In the following section, we will briefly review a sample of the research describing individual characteristics commonly associated with resilience, including temperament, intellectual development, self-esteem, internal locus of control, mastery, and social support, and explore the relational aspects of these characteristics. Our discussion will conclude with a case example and recommendations for strengthening resilience.

A RELATIONALLY TEMPERED TEMPERAMENT

For many years researchers have explored the internal, relatively stable, individual trait of temperament and its association with a child's ability to be resilient (Rutter, 1978; Werner & Smith, 1982). In their groundbreaking, 40-year study of 698 multi- and mixed-racial children living in adverse conditions on the Hawaiian Island of Kauai, Emma Werner and her colleagues (1982) found that boys described as "good natured" and girls described as "cuddly" were more resilient than other children. While some researchers might focus their investigations on describing the temperament of resilient children, an RCT perspective would suggest that researchers should examine the relational implications of temperament. Michael Rutter (1989) did just that. He found that children with difficult temperaments were twice as likely to be the targets of parental criticism. His research suggests that a child's temperament either protects or puts a child at risk because of its positive or negative impact on the *parent-child relationship.* In other words, a child's temperament affects the child's and the parent's ability to engage in relationships, i.e., temperament tempers relationships.

Based on Rutter and Werner's observations, one might conclude that good-natured boys and perhaps cuddly girls would be the most resilient children and children with difficult temperaments would be the least resilient. However, RCT encourages us to take a broader view and examine how the social/cultural context interacts with a child's temperament and his or her relational opportunities. One study of East African Masai children living in severe drought conditions found that the children with more difficult temperaments were more likely to survive (de Vries, 1984). Noting that Masai culture values assertiveness, the researchers theorized that the difficult (assertive) children were more able to access the relational resources they needed to survive severe hardships. This one example illustrates how differences in temperament influence one's relational opportunities within a specific social/cultural context. Moving beyond efforts to precisely describe the temperaments of resilient and nonresilient children, an RCT perspective would suggest that researchers could do more to describe *in depth and in detail* the optimal relational practices and cultural conditions that promote resilience in children with disparate temperaments. This would help clinicians identify the most helpful relational skills needed in the parent-child relationship to strengthen the resilience of the child *and the parent*.

CONNECTING INTELLECTUAL AND RELATIONAL DEVELOPMENT

The literature and research on resilience clearly indicate that individuals with greater intelligence are more resilient, yet the reason for this advantage is not clear. Ann Masten and her colleagues (Masten, 1994, 2001; Masten, Best, & Garmezy, 1990) propose a number of explanations. It could be that individuals with greater intelligence are more able to discern danger and find escape routes, may have educational advantages when compared to others, or may have more capable parents. Exploring a relational view of intellectual development, Daniel Siegle (1999) emphasizes that interpersonal relationships are the central source of experience that influences the brain's development. Neural pathways in the brain are activated by experiential opportunities provided to children through relational engagement, which results in "strengthening existing connections or creating new connections" (Ibid., p. 13). Siegle observes that "Interpersonal experience thus plays a special organizing role in determining the development of brain structure early in life and the ongoing emergence of brain function throughout the life-span" (Ibid., p. 24). Hence, "human connections create neuronal connections" (Ibid., p. 85).

Siegle emphasizes that relationships play a key role in optimizing an individual's intelligence and consequently their ability to be resilient. For therapists, efforts to strengthen a client's resilience could involve proactively encouraging the client's participation in relationships that provide experiences that increase intellectual opportunities and stimulation. While this may be an obvious endeavor for therapists working with children or adolescents, therapists working with adults and seniors may find this way of strengthening resilience highly beneficial for reducing the diminished cognitive functions often associated with aging (Crose, 1997).

FROM SELF-ESTEEM TO SENSE OF WORTH

Self-esteem is probably the most commonly known and widely accepted internal personality trait associated with resilience (Dumont & Provost, 1999). Nevertheless, scholars of RCT draw into question the conceptualization of this characteristic. Judith Jordan (1994) observed that Western-European society has tended to describe self-esteem based on the cultural values of individual achievement and self-sufficiency, as opposed to collaboration and connection. Consequently, a person's self-esteem may depend upon hierarchical comparisons in which one perpetually strives to feel superior to others in one way or another. Developing "healthy" self-esteem within this context becomes a competitive exercise to demonstrate that one's achievements are better than someone else's. Furthermore, those who do not participate in this method of building self-esteem, or those who do not subscribe to the dominant cultural values of self-sufficiency, may be perceived as having lower self-esteem.

Bernadette Gray-Little's (2000) research illustrates this point. For many years black children were thought to have lower self-esteem than white children do. This presumption followed a 1947 study in which black children were asked to choose between two dolls that were identical except one was black and the other white. When the black children chose the white doll, the researchers interpreted this result as a sign of black children's low self-esteem. Gray-Little refuted this conclusion generalized from this study and from similar research by examining over 261 studies of over half-a-million children. Her careful review of the research indicated that black children had at least as high levels of self-esteem as white children, and in some cases their self-esteem was even higher. According to Gray-Little, research like the 1947 study may be indicative of how a racial group is valued in society, but it is not indicative of the level of black children's self-esteem. Additionally, Gray-Little challenges the view that self-esteem is built on a ladder of individual achievement, noting that, "Self-esteem is determined by our interactions with people significant to us personally" (Fletcher, 2000). Her relational view is supported by other research showing that self-esteem correlates with a child's closeness to his or her mother, and increased closeness is associated with higher self-esteem (Burnett & Demnar, 1996). Others have shown that adolescent self-esteem is positively correlated with involvement with family, community, and one's neighborhood (Dumont & Provost, 1999).

Taking a broader cultural perspective, Yvonne Jenkins (1993) proposes that individualistic conceptualizations of self-esteem may have limited relevance to people of color. Jenkins suggests that a group-centered, relational understanding of esteem is more useful for understanding the esteem of some people of color. She calls this *social esteem*. A person's social esteem is formed through association with a group-related identity that values "interdependence, affiliation, and collaterality" (p. 55). Jenkins observes that, *"for collective societies, group esteem is practi-*

cally synonymous with the Anglo-centric conceptualizations of self-esteem" (p. 55). For populations in which the unit of operation is the family, the group, or the collective society, social esteem may be an essential part of healthy psychosocial development and part of one's ability to cope with adversity.

Jean Baker Miller (1986) offers another alternative to what is known as self-esteem. She suggests that it may be more useful to think of this concept in terms of "sense of worth." Sense of worth grows through engagement in relationships in which people feel known and valued–relationships in which the other person "conveys attention to, and recognition of, our experience" (p. 6). Miller (1991) believes that the concept of a "self" as it has been formulated in Western culture reinforces a sense of psychological separation from others (p. 25). Perhaps the separate-self connotation embedded in the popular notion of self-esteem inspires efforts to build esteem by elevating oneself over or by diminishing others, which can become an insatiable pursuit. Rather than something one earns at the expense of others, Jean Baker Miller's notion of sense of worth is an outcome of participating in growth-fostering relationships, which benefits all who participate in the relationship. Furthermore, a relationally based sense of worth, knowing that one matters to someone else, as opposed to an achievement-based sense of self-esteem, may be another essential reservoir of energy strengthening one's ability to be resilient. Clearly this is demonstrated in effective and healing therapy relationships.

FROM INTERNAL CONTROL TO MUTUAL EMPOWERMENT

A number of researchers have identified internal locus of control (ILOC) as another individual characteristic associated with resilience (Masten, Best, & Garmezy, 1990; Werner & Smith, 1982). According to a textbook definition by Roediger and his colleagues (1991):

> Children who take responsibility for their own successes and failures are said to have an internal locus of control. (p. 352)

This definition focuses on one's individual responsibility in response to individual experience, but it does not account for the impact of racism, sexism, heterosexism, or other forms of discrimination that can influence one's ability to take responsibility for successes or failures. For instance, it may be easier to establish an internal sense of control when one is a member of a social group in society that is viewed as the norm or ideal, i.e., the dominant group (Miller, 1976). Members of dominant groups are recipients of unearned advantages that facilitate their successes and mitigate their failures (McIntosh, 1989). As a result, it may be easier for these individuals to develop an internal sense of control, easier for them to take responsibility, because they are living in a society that encourages their success and cushions their failures. Furthermore, persuading subordinate groups that they should have a greater internal locus of control–i.e., they *should* feel responsible for their lack of success as well as their failures–may work to the advantage of the dominant group. Encouraging subordinates to attribute their lack of success and failures to some form of internal deficiency, e.g., lack of ILOC, distracts them from questioning external practices that impede their success and encourage their failure.

A recent study exploring the stress resilience of white and black children helps us rethink our understanding of ILOC (Magnus, Cowen, Wyman, Fagen, & Work, 1999). This study compared stress resilient (SR) white and black children with stress affected (SA) white and black children. As expected, the study showed that SR white children had a greater sense of internal locus of control than the SA white children; however, no significant difference in ILOC was found between the SR and the SA black children. These results led the researchers to theorize that black families may de-emphasize ILOC because it encourages a false belief that one can or should be able to control pervasive, socially constructed adversities such as racism and other forms of discrimination.

Rather than using the language of internal or external control, RCT describes the relational phenomenon of mutual empowerment, which is a two-way dynamic process that grows out of participation in responsive, mutually empathic relationships (Miller & Stiver, 1997). Mutual empowerment is a sense that both (or all) people in the relationship have the ability to influence their experience and the relationship, and are able to take action on behalf of themselves and others. Using the construct of mutual empowerment rather than internal, individual control, researchers could explore whether or not people are more resilient when they are engaged in responsive relationships where they feel they have the capacity to influence their experience. RCT would suggest, and clinical practice supports, that mutual empowerment is an essential healing ingredient in the therapy relationship, which makes it possible for clients to overcome hardships, turmoil, and adversities (Jordan, Kaplan, Miller, Stiver, & Surrey, 1991; Miller, 1988, 2002).

FROM MASTERY TO COMPETENCE THROUGH CONNECTION

The literature on resilience often uses the term "mastery" to refer to the instrumental behavior one develops to conquer a challenging situation or task (Masten, Best, & Garmezy, 1991). RCT scholar Judith Jordan (1999) questions the use of this term because of the tacit connotation associated with the word "master." Jordan explains that "'to master' is to reduce to subjection, to get the better of, to break, to tame" (p. 1-2). Consequently:

> mastery implicit in most models of competence creates enormous conflict for many people, especially women and other marginalized groups, people who have not traditionally been "the masters." (Ibid., p. 2)

Jordan goes on to propose that "competence" may be a more useful, less contaminated term for describing the development of skills that contribute to one's ability to be resilient. Moreover, Jordan notes that competence is not developed in isolation; competence grows through connection. It evolves through engagement in relationships that support, encourage, and inspire our efforts to overcome challenges and hardships.

Many relationships can contribute to the development of competence, e.g., relationships with parents, family members, teachers, mentors, peers, supervisors, employers, etc. For example, according to Ann Masten and her colleagues (1990), parents can strengthen their children's sense of competence by:

1. Being a model of effective action for their children.
2. Providing their children with opportunities to experience competence, and
3. Verbally affirming the competence of their children, by affirming their children's ability to develop new skills and utilize these skills effectively.

Therapists play a key role in encouraging and affirming the competence of their clients. Often those who enter therapy have lost their sense of efficacy as well as their confidence in themselves and their relationships. Within a mutually empathic, growth-fostering relational environment, clients can rebuild and reclaim their sense of competence to address the challenges they must face in their lives.

FROM SOCIAL SUPPORT TO AUTHENTIC CONNECTION

Social support has been well documented as a factor that contributes to one's ability to be resilient (Atkins, Kaplan, & Toshima, 1991; Belle, 1987; Ganellen & Blaney, 1984; Ornish, 1997). Of all the constructs discussed thus far, social support is obviously the most relational. However, from the perspective of RCT, social support has significant limitations. Social support is most often described in the research as a *one-way, unidirectional* form of relating, or something that one gets from others (Fiore, Becker, & Coppel, 1983). In addition, researchers know that some experiences of social support can have negative consequences (Belle, 1982).

In contrast to the one-way notion of social support, RCT emphasizes the *two-way, bi-directional* nature of relationships, that is, the two-way, growth-promoting quality of relating known as *connection* (Jordan, 1992). Connection is cultivated in relationships through the practice of mutual empathy, relational responsiveness, mutual empowerment, authenticity, and movement toward mutuality (Jordan, 1986). The two-way nature of growth-promoting connection has been a central premise of RCT throughout its 25-year development, and recently more researchers have begun to note the importance of understanding connection and the bi-directional nature of relationships that foster resilience (Blum, McNeely, & Rinehart 2002; Masten, 2001; Masten, Hubbard, Gest, Tellegen, Garmezy, & Ramirez, 1999; Resnick et al., 1997).

Renée Spencer's review of the research describes the evidence indicating that children who have at least one supportive relationship (connection) with an adult can achieve good outcomes despite severe hardships. These hardships include parental mental illness (Rutter, 1979), separation from a parent (Rutter, 1971), marital discord (Rutter, 1971), divorcing parents (Wallerstein & Kelly, 1980), poverty (Garmezy, 1991), maltreatment (Cicchetti, 1989), and multifaceted or a combination of risk factors (Seifer et al., 1996). Michael Resnick's (1997) large-scale study of 12,000 adolescents found that *a sense of connection* (e.g., to parents, family members, or other adults) reduces the risk that a child will experience substance abuse, violence, depression, suicidal behavior, and early sexual activity regardless of race, ethnicity, socioeconomic status, or family structure. This challenges the traditional view that healthy adolescents need to separate from the important relationships in their lives. In fact, severing "apron strings" may be putting children at greater risk for developing psychological or behavioral problems. The turmoil often associated with adolescence may not be a signal for separation, (a.k.a. independence), but a signal to parents and adults to find better ways to stay connected to their children as they grow and change.

Connection appears to be particularly important for children in school. Robert Blum and his colleagues (2002) surveyed over 90,000 adolescents from 80 different communities during one academic year and found that students who felt connected in school were less likely to use cigarettes, alcohol, or drugs; less likely to engage in early sexual activity, violence, or become pregnant; and less likely to experience emotional distress. The researchers observed that, "when students feel they are a part of school, say they are treated fairly by teachers, and feel close to people at school, they are healthier and are more likely to succeed" (p. 2). Sadly, the data also showed that 31 percent of students do not feel connected at school.

A sense of connection is also essential for adults. In his national analysis of social connectedness, Harvard Professor Robert Putnam (2000) concluded that studies ". . . have established beyond reasonable doubt that social connectedness is one of the most powerful determinants of our well being" (p. 326). In fact, according to Putnam, ". . . happiness is best predicted by the breadth and depth of one's social connections" (p. 332). In another example of research, Berkman and Syme (1979) found that men and women who were married, who had contact with close friends and relatives, or who had informal or formal group associations had "lower mortality rates than respondents lacking such connections" (p. 188).

Connection may be especially important for promoting women's resilience. Research by Taylor and her colleagues (2000) proposes that women utilize a *tend-and-befriend* response to stress rather than a flight-or-fight response. These researchers believe the fight/flight response is inhibited in women by neurobiological processes that mitigate their feelings of fear, diminish their sympathetic nervous system activity, and stimulate their care-taking and affiliative behavior. In response to threat, women may engage in care-giving activities or affiliative activities to protect themselves and the important people in their lives (e.g., children). This analysis is supported by other research showing that women are more likely to draw upon social support in times of stress, maintain close relationships with female friends, and engage in social groups more often than men (Belle, 1987). The tend-and-befriend theory is an interesting reformulation of responses to threat. However, on a note of caution, more research needs to be completed to explore larger applications of this model. For instance, Taylor and her colleagues (2000) state that the model may also apply to some aspects of men's behavior, but this research has yet to be conducted.

Therapists have known for a long time that social support can be helpful, but RCT helps us understand that it is the *quality* of the connection that makes social support beneficial. Social support that fosters mutual empathy, mutual empowerment, and authentic connection can strengthen a client's ability to respond effectively to difficult and devastating situations.

THE CASE OF JENNIFER AND JULIE: STRENGTHENING RESILIENCE THROUGH RELATIONSHIPS

Sisters Jennifer and Julie were recently placed in a pre-adoptive home after many months in foster care. Two years before, they were removed from their birth home because of the abuse and neglect they experienced at the hands of drug-addicted parents whose parental rights were eventually terminated. With the help of therapy, Jennifer and Julie had made great strides to deal with the trauma they had experienced in their biological home and they were looking forward to being adopted into a permanent home that was recently identified for them. To facilitate this process, Jennifer, Julie, and their pre-adoptive parents were referred to an adoption support program offered at a community mental health agency where I became their therapist.

From the start, I noted that Julie and Jennifer were very different from each other. Eight-year-old Jennifer was described by previous social workers as a bright, attractive, affable, attentive child with a pleasant temperament, a positive self-esteem, and few obvious signs of her history of trauma and neglect. She excelled at school and had many friends. On the other hand, 11-year-old Julie was considered the "troubled child" with a difficult, emotionally liable temperament and borderline intellectual abilities. She was highly distractible, impulsive, and hyperactive with a chronically disheveled appearance (e.g., torn or dirty clothes, uncombed, unkempt hair, and poor personal hygiene). She had few friends and did poorly in school. Using an individual strength perspective, one would say that Jennifer had the most resilience for adapting to an adoptive home while Julie faced daunting obstacles. These disparate sisters were placed in the home of "Janice" and "Jim," two mature, first-time parents who hoped to offer the girls a permanent home.

Clinicians who work in field know that the majority of adoptions of older children fail, so I felt I had realistic concerns about the success of this adoption. In the week before the family came to see me, the parents had become highly exasperated by Julie's behavior. They were concerned that they would "never be able to manage all of her problems and antics." They confessed that they would be tempted to adopt Jennifer without Julie, but recognized that this would be a crushing blow to the girls. Fortunately, these parents were very eager and open to working with me and continued to hope that they could find a way to provide these girls with a loving home.

My goal working with these parents was to help them foster the relational development of their new family, utilizing the principles and practices of RCT. This meant working with the family to build their relational strengths and skills to be resilient throughout the process of forming a new family unit. This process began with encouraging the parents to take a relational-contextual view of Jennifer and Julie's behavior rather than an individualistic view. In other words, encouraging the parents to examine Jennifer and Julie's behavior in the context of their relational history and experience.

For example, a relational perspective eventually allowed the parents to consider the possibility that Julie may have developed her difficult behaviors to ensure her survival in response to living in a severely abusive and neglectful birth home. This relational analysis and awareness of Julie's experience and difficult behaviors permitted the parents to overcome their temptation to target Julie for excessive criticism for being internally deficient or damaged, and inspired the parents to find loving, creative, and effective ways to help Julie manage her behavior. Greater relational awareness also helped the parents notice and avoid negatively comparing Julie's intellectual abilities with her younger sister's. Instead, they became proactive in their efforts to get Julie the special resources and support to be more successful in school. The parents also found ways to help Julie develop a circle of friends beyond her relationship with her sister.

Interestingly, as the parents gained greater confidence in their ability to be responsive to Julie's challenging behavior, Julie gained greater confidence in herself and in her new family. These are symptoms of the relational resilience growing among the family members. In particular, there were many changes in Julie's behavior. Most notably Julie's hyperactive, distractible, impulsive behavior began to recede significantly at home and at school. In addition, Julie's increased sense of worth, derived from the love of her new parents went hand-in-hand with her attentiveness to maintaining her personal appearance and hygiene. Julie's transformation was so pronounced that her former therapist did not recognize Julie as the same client she worked with two years earlier.

As Julie's behaviors began to change, it became clear to me and the parents that Jennifer's "ideal" behavior was largely part of her special strategy of survival (Stiver, 1992), adopted in response to her history of living in an abusive environment. Once again, a relational analysis helped us see that Jennifer took on the role of the "responsible child" in order to take care of her difficult sister. She was a parentified child, a role that came at the price of being authentic, carefree, spontaneous, and playful. Eventually, Jennifer began to see that her adoptive parents were able to take care of Julie and constructively respond to her behavior. Based on this, Jennifer gained confidence in her relationship with her adoptive parents, trusting that they could be responsible and loving parents. This allowed Jennifer to relinquish much of her adult-like behavior and become the lively, spontaneous, sometimes mischievous child you would expect.

In this situation, all members of this family developed greater resilience through relationships. The sisters became more resilient through their relationships with the parents, which allowed both Julie and Jennifer to relinquish old strategies of survival. The parents become more resilient through their relationship with the therapist and others who supported their efforts to create a loving family. The parents' successful efforts to strengthen their new family's development and resilience were obvious to all who knew this family. Eventually, Janice and Jim were honored with a special award from a statewide organization for being models of outstanding parenting.

RELATIONAL WAYS TO STRENGTHEN RESILIENCE

This article proposes that resilience is strengthened through relationships, specifically, mutually empathic, mutually empowering, growth-fostering relationships. This view is supported by a review of the research examining individual characteristics commonly associated with resilience and describing the relational aspects of these characteristics. Taking a relational view moves the concept of resilience beyond the intrinsic toughness model, in which resilience is available to a few inherently lucky individuals, to understanding that greater resilience is available to us all through relationships. This opens the way to new sources of hope and courage as we individually and collectively face unpredictable threats while living in a risky world.

The practice of effective therapy is often about strengthening a client's ability to be resilient through relationship. In particular, a relational therapist is attuned to the connections and disconnections within the therapeutic process and in the client's life that promote or impede the client's ability to overcome adversities. Working together, the client and therapist can develop a "tool kit" of relational ways to enhance and strengthen the resilience of the client as well as the resilience of the therapeutic relationship. The following is a beginning list of relational ways a therapist may enhance the resilience of her or his clients:

1. Explore the client's access to relationships that support his/her ability to be resilient, particularly relationships that are responsive to his/her unique individual characteristics (e.g., temperament, intelligence, etc.).
2. Help clients identify, establish, and expand relationships that contribute to their ability to be resilient, relationships characterized by mutual empathy, mutual empowerment, and responsiveness (i.e., growth-fostering relationships).
3. Encourage clients to identify and seek relationships that stimulate and support their intellectual development as well as contribute to their learning opportunities (e.g., mentors, teachers, supervisors, etc.).
4. Help clients to enhance their sense of worth through engagement in meaningful relationships (e.g., with family, friends, community groups, etc.) rather than through competitive achievements or personal comparisons.
5. Show clients that they have an impact on the therapy relationship as well as on other relationships, which will strengthen their ability to take positive action on behalf of themselves, others, and their relationships (Miller, 2002). Encourage clients to find opportunities to enhance their sense of competence and verbally convince them of their competence by providing praise, guidance, and/or constructive feedback (Masten, 1999).
6. Use moments of conflict in therapy to show the client that disagreements can be opportunities to enhance relational authenticity and strengthen confidence in connection, thus increasing the client's relational resilience in therapy and in other relationships.

7. Explore the client's opportunities to create more connections through peer groups, community groups, *mutual-help* groups, or formal or informal mutual support groups.
8. Examine ways the client can make meaningful contributions to others through community action, community service, social action, mentoring, teaching, etc.

These suggestions can be summarized as finding more and more ways to expand our clients' experiences of growth-fostering relationships, relationships characterized by mutual empathy, mutual empowerment, mutuality, zest, clarity, increasing sense of worth, and a desire for more connection (Miller & Stiver, 1997). But, these are not only good recommendations for clients in therapy, these are good recommendations for *all* of us. In this risky world, all of us can benefit from proactively identifying relationships that promote our resilience, our intellectual development, our sense of worth, our sense of competence, our sense of empowerment, and, most importantly, our sense of connection. Because *strengthening resilience is all about relationships.*

REFERENCES

Brock, R. N. (1993). Journeys by heart: A christology of erotic power. New York: Crossroads Press.

Dorn, J., Flack, R., & Jackson, J. (1971). Go Up, Moses. [Recorded by Flack, R.]. On Quiet Fire [CD]. New York: Atlantic Records.

Fischer, K. (1999). Transforming fire: Women using anger creatively. Mahwah, NJ: Paulist Press.

Fletcher, J., Jordan, J., & Miller, J. (2000). Women and the workplace: Applications of psychodynamic theory. The American Journal of Psychoanalysis, 60(3), 243-261.

hooks, b. (2000). Feminist theory: From margin to center (2nd ed.). Cambridge, MA: South End Press.

Janeway, E. (1980). Powers of the weak. New York: Knopf.

Jordan, J. V. (1991). Empathy and self boundaries. In J. Jordan, A. Kaplan, J. Miller, I. Stiver, & J. Surrey (Eds.). Women's growth in connection. New York: Guilford Press.

Jordan, J. V. (2002, April). Courage in connection: Working with vulnerability. Paper presented at the Harvard Learning from Women Conference co-sponsored by Harvard Medical School/Cambridge Hospital and the Jean Baker Miller Training Institute, Boston, MA.

Kollias, K. (1975). Class realities: Creating a new power base. Quest, 1(3), 28-43.

Miller, J. B. (1986). Toward a new psychology of women (2nd ed.). Boston: Beacon Press.

Miller, J. B. (1991). Women and power. In J. Jordan, A. Kaplan, J. Miller, I. Stiver, & J. Surrey (Eds.). Women's growth in connection. New York: Guilford Press.

Rubin, H. (1998). The princessa: Machiavelli for women. New York: Dell Books.

Stiver, I. (1991). Work inhibitions in women. In J. Jordan, A. Kaplan, J. Miller, I. Stiver, & J. Surrey (Eds.). Women's growth in connection. New York: Guilford Press.

Thomas, D. (2002). Unpublished symposium comments. Harvard University, February 6, 2002.

Walker, A. (1979). Janie Crawford in Good night, Willie Lee, I'll See You in the Morning. San Diego: Harvest/Harcourt Brace and Janovich.

Williamson, M. (1996). A return to love: Reflections on the principles of a course in miracles. New York: HarperCollins.

When Racism Gets Personal: Toward Relational Healing

Maureen Walker

SUMMARY. In a culture that stratifies human differences, it is inevitable that anxiety about difference would be the source of much suffering. The power distortions that lie at the root of this suffering are manifest in relationships, from the most tangential to those that are deeply intimate. Moreover, the anxieties endemic to a race-based culture have the potential to thwart our most earnest efforts to make and maintain good connection. To adopt the feminist perspective, that the personal is political, is to acknowledge that no relationship can remain unscathed when power and value are differentially accorded based on racial group membership.

Three examples from clinical practice will be used to illustrate how racial anxiety impedes movement toward authenticity, mutuality, and empowerment in intimate relationships. In these examples, three biracial women who identify as black navigate the racial stratifications that contaminate the inevitable conflicts in their relationships with parents, mentors, and lovers. Because of the multilayered anxieties stemming from living and loving in a racially stratified culture, conflicts, which might otherwise be the source of growth and deeper connection, become

---

Maureen Walker, PhD, is Director of Program Development, JBMTI; Associate Director of Support Services, Harvard Business School; in private practice for psychotherapy and multicultural consultation, Cambridge, MA; and co-editor of *How Connections Heal* and *The Complexity of Connection*.

rigidified and immobilizing. In addition to examining the debilitating impact of racial anxiety, the presentation will highlight the relational processes that facilitate healing, resilience, and mutual empowerment.

INTRODUCTION

Everyday encounters bring us face to face with the complexities of living, working, and loving in a racially diverse world. We encounter this complexity in the changing arenas and shifting alignments of love and work. In most instances, we think of these changes as social progress. However, underlying this apparent progress is a social-historical trauma, the sequel of which can erupt–seemingly unbidden–at any given moment. It was within this context of complexity that about five years ago I came to know a precocious, young woman whom I will call Lauren. Lauren described herself as biracial: the daughter of an African American father who had grown up during the forties and fifties in rural Arkansas and a white Jewish mother who had grown up in suburban Seattle in the sixties. The culture that shaped Lauren's parents was far different from the social spaces that Lauren inhabited. Unlike her parents, Lauren grew up in a time and place where legal barriers to the corridors of commerce and education had been dissolved for racial minorities. Legislative prohibitions against interracial unions had been repealed for the most part. Lauren's was a world where the social spaces reflected an ethnic and economic diversity unfamiliar to earlier generations, and the people she called friends and family were multi-colored and multi-cultured. For all of its cultural richness and social privilege, Lauren experienced her world as stifling and constricted. In one of our therapy sessions, she commented: "When my father accuses me of thinking about race too much, but blames my mother for not talking about it at all; when my mother can't understand the part of me that is black–that's when racism really gets personal."

In a culture that stratifies human difference, that systematically rank orders human beings according to their racial group membership, it is inevitable that anxiety about racial difference would be the source of much human suffering. The resulting power distortions give rise to anxieties that manifest themselves in our relationships–from the most tangential to the most intimate. These are the anxieties endemic to a race-based culture, and they have the potential to thwart our best efforts to make and maintain good connection. In situational relationships–whether in the context of work or a commercial transaction–racial anxiety can trigger unease and generate a stultifying awkwardness. In more intimate relationships–whether among parents and spouses, mentors and lovers, or colleagues and friends–racial anxiety can stifle authenticity and inhibit mutuality. In any relationship, multi-layered anxieties deriving from working and loving in a racially stratified culture can contaminate the everyday conflicts, which might otherwise be the source of creative movement and deeper connection.

Poet and activist Audre Lorde once said that it is not our differences that separate us. It is rather our refusal to recognize those differences; it is rather our refusal to examine the distortions that result from misnaming those differences (1984). The cultural tendency to frame difference in dichotomous and oppositional terms also gives rise to relational distortion. To paraphrase Lorde, this culture offers few models of mutual and authentic engagement across difference. What we experience as racial separation is often caused by our refusal to acknowledge the impact of the distortions upon human behavior and expectation. This refusal to engage the resulting complexity pushes us into chronic disconnection. It plunges us into an immobilizing anxiety that betrays our yearning for connection.

Psychotherapists have a unique opportunity to confront and examine the racial anxieties that perpetuate distortion and disconnection. The Relational-Cultural Model provides a critical standpoint from which to engage three questions. First, how do we understand the genesis and the manifestation of racial anxiety in relationship? Second, how does this anxiety shape behavior and relational expectation? And third, how do we make creative use of racial anxiety to foster resilience and reconnection? In exploring these three questions, I have found it helpful to use a model proposed by psychotherapist and author Robert Gerzon, whose tripartite model of anxiety provides a useful framework for understanding the personalized experience of historical racial trauma. The historical trauma of racism translates into cognitive-emotive experiences that may be described as natural anxiety, toxic anxiety, and sacred anxiety. This three-part model of anxiety clarifies that processes of disconnection can thwart the most earnest efforts to engage across racial difference. Because anxiety constricts the range of relational movement and possibility, the cultural trauma of racism may significantly undermine the most personal relationships.

Few people would argue with the philosophers who have asserted over the ages that life is difficult. Natural anxiety is defined as a response of awareness to that difficulty, as recognition of our inevitable limitations (Gerzon, 1999). Natural anxiety is an expression of the uncertainty and ambivalence that checks our expectation for, and our movement in relationship. With the dissolution of visible and legislated barriers to cross-racial contact, the social cues that guide relationship have become increasingly ambiguous. There appears to be more relational space within which to navigate. However, because of what anthropologist Karen Brodkin (1999) has called the binary system of racial categorization, it is possible, as some have said, for black and white citizens to sit in the same theater, but each see a very different movie. In other words, in spite of the ambiguity, the categories remain intact–though somewhat more mystified. When relational expectation is defined by a racial binary, the enlargement of the socio-cultural arena may lead not to fuller or expanded connection, but to diminished authenticity. As one Latina corporate executive commented, "Being promoted in this organization simply means having to function in more and more spaces where I can't be myself." Faced with the racial conundrum of demarcation and ambiguity, natural anxiety is a reasonable response. Natural anxiety is a natural response to navigating through a relational fog.

LAUREN'S DILEMMA

I can think of no better example of a relational fog and its attendant anxiety than that provided by nineteen-year-old Lauren. Once when talking about her lackluster middle school performance, Lauren recalled a game that was directed by her eighth grade social studies teacher. It was called "The Plantation Game." The object of the game was to buy and sell slaves and see who could have the most profitable plantation; the teacher's objective was to demonstrate the economic motivations behind slavery and to prove that racial prejudice was consequent to, but not the cause of, race slavery. Although her memory was mercifully fuzzy, Lauren could not recall any lessons about the brutality of slavery. She remembered some conversation about people whom she dubbed "celebrity slaves like Frederick Douglass," but not about slaves in general, as if they were actually human beings. Lauren described herself as the only "black-half black" student in this elite prep school classroom.

She recalled getting up and walking around the class bartering and feeling really awful. She went from hating the teacher to liking him to hating herself to believing that the teacher was her friend and would never hurt her to concluding that he had horribly betrayed and humiliated her. She said: "Race was a topic never broached in my home. When I was eleven, I didn't know anything about racism, I didn't know about black or white, but I *did* know that I was different in a way that was not positive." She continued: "I knew something needed to be said, but I didn't want to be the one to say 'it'; I didn't even know what 'it' was; and I didn't want anyone else to bring it up because I *was* the only black-half black student in the room."

She remembered that the teacher was very popular and the other students all seemed to enjoy the assignment. Clearly, in her mind, something was wrong with what *she* was feeling. Lauren's experience is totally consistent with the observation that the person violated will often feel at fault for the disconnection (Miller, 1988). Lauren had three other very clear recollections about this incident: that when she finally told her parents they were furious; that her mother promised to speak with the teacher at the end of the school year; and that life in the eighth grade was never the same. So anxious was she about the threat of exclusion *and* the indignity of inclusion, that she placed herself in a kind of academic and emotional limbo. Not able to extricate and not willing to engage, she remained safely on the margins–as she said, "doing just enough to get a B- without really trying."

To ensure her psychological survival, Lauren employed various strategies of disconnection and dissemblance–not only in school, but with her parents as well. To the extent that we come to know and grow ourselves through action in relationship, Lauren could not know herself, nor could she authentically represent that which she knew.

In many of our sessions, a great part of my work was to hold Lauren's yearning for connection with her mother, a yearning so fraught with anxiety that she could barely tolerate it. At various times, Lauren and her mother would engage in verbal "power over" struggles that they perceived as attempts to communicate. In these conversations, each would try to convert the other to her point of view on a given subject. It was often the case that the content of the conversation was far less important than the intent: to change or somehow unsettle the other person. In other words, conversations were contests that they each wanted to win. The inevitable outcome would be long periods of silence between them, as both women had well-honed strategies for disconnection.

Lauren would then disappear into MTV, while her mother would disappear into depressive behaviors.

When Lauren recounted these episodes in therapy–criticizing her mother's inadequacy and inaccessibility–it was important to hold the yearning by both empathizing with her distress and by naming some true thing about positive aspects of their relationship (Stiver, personal communication, 1998). For example, I would often say something about their desire to be visible to and be known by each other. At various times, it was useful to reframe their conflicts as "tenacious efforts to create mutuality." Indeed, what each woman wanted was to know that she could have an impact on the other. Each woman yearned deeply for reassurance that the other would not abandon her. Both women were terrified by their yearning. Lauren's mother was profoundly threatened by the vehemence with which her daughter undertook the so-called task of separation: a task rendered even more threatening by the ever visible racial divide between them. Lauren, for her part, needed to know that she could move and be moved by her mother–and that in the movement, she would remain safe.

On one occasion when they were "communicating," Lauren gave her mother a fairly detailed account of her sexual history. Her mother responded quite predictably–she got sick and went to bed. Although Lauren recounted her mother's horrified response as a personal victory because it was further proof of mother's ineptness, she was nonetheless quite pained by this encounter. After we worked through the first level of the narrative, which included painstaking efforts to name her feelings, I asked how was she *hoping* her mother would respond. Lauren answered by stating what she expected. "But what were you *hoping* for?"

Eventually, and with a great deal of difficulty, Lauren was able to say that she wished her mother had been able to talk with her about the raw pain and mocking emptiness of her adolescent years–that she wished her mother could have held her. Because of repeated ruptures in their relationship, Lauren had come to associate her hopes and her yearning with shame, disappointment, and unsafe vulnerability. One important relational skill for Lauren to develop was more respect for her hopes and more empathy for her disappointments.

From this place of emotional expansion, Lauren was able to recollect more positive images of herself with her mother. For example, she remembered how she and her mother would hold hands walking down the street, and how they would laugh uproariously at the quizzical looks they would get from onlookers who didn't understand this expression of tenderness and affection between two women, of apparently different race and age. From time to time, she could also express empathy with her mother's weariness and understand her wariness in the face of racial difference. In other words, she was occasionally able to practice the critical distinction between anticipatory empathy and self-abnegation. From a place of connection with her own feeling-thoughts, she was able to tolerate feeling with another.

Clinical Post-Scripts

Because the cultural context of therapy was one that placed undue emphasis on maternal inadequacy as the source of clinical problems, it was especially important to hold and honor Lauren's barely articulated yearning for her mother. Furthermore, it was important to be mindful of the racial anxieties that surrounded the therapy, anxieties with the potential to exacerbate the ruptures created by a patriarchal culture that tends to devalue and blame mothers and daughters. For that reason, a clinical imperative was to mindfully refrain from tacit competition with Lauren's mother (as we therapists are sometimes prone to do).

A significant part of Lauren's sub-textual narrative was that her life would have been better had her mother been black. As an African American therapist, it was important to avoid colluding with these seductive fantasies, thus establishing myself as "good mother." Second, some would suggest that many of the conflicts Lauren described were typical struggles of adolescence. While that observation is probably true, it is equally true that the anxieties and fears endemic to a racially stratified culture tainted these struggles. When relational images are conditioned by a racialized culture, race not only becomes the default explanation for any disconnection–it also exploits the inevitable tensions and processes of relational movement.

Often toxic anxiety sits at the root of racialized conflict. As Gerzon (1998) observed, toxic anxiety results from habitually suppressing thoughts, desires, and memories. In the binary system of racial ranking, suppression is standard operating procedure. As Miller pointed out, rigid ranking generates power distortions that trigger conflict, and simultaneously seek to suppress it (1986). The inevitable anxiety centers on past hurts, both individual and collective. It consists of intergenerational memory on the one hand and historical amnesia on the other. This anxiety can reduce potentially productive interactions to ritualized performance. When it remains unacknowledged and unexplored, racial anxiety may rise in toxic form–sabotaging desire for connection.

SARA'S DILEMMA

An example of racial anxiety turned toxic can be seen in the dilemma that Sara presented in therapy. Sara described herself as biracial and lesbian. Her primary complaint was feeling sadness and guilt about her inability to sustain satisfying relationships. She said that she had been in many therapies before and that this time, she specifically wanted to work with someone familiar with the Relational-Cultural Model. When I asked how she hoped *this* work would be different, she said that "I know something is missing inside me, and I think it's making me mess up my relationships." As we got to know each other over the next several weeks, I learned that Sara was the daughter of a biracial mother who had married a Jamaican man while still a teenager. She was quite young when Sara was born, and by Sara's account, totally overwhelmed by the motherhood experience. What Sara remembers most about her early childhood was her mother's passivity. As she described the relationship: "I learned at an early age to have no respect for her at all." At various points in the therapy, she would talk about her mother with total disdain; her favorite descriptor was "useless." In fact, she had spent most of her 29 years thinking of her mother as intellectually and characterologically inferior to herself. It became apparent that this expressed contempt was in fact a strategy of disconnection used to disguise her yearning for connection with her mother and to assuage the distress of having concluded that such connection was beyond reach.

Although Sara described herself and her mother as biracial, she thought of her mother as white, and in many ways attributed their disconnection to their racial difference. As she put it, "my mother was *totally mystified* by my hair." Further conversation revealed Sara's sense that her mother was certainly frustrated, and probably disapproving of her hair. For her part, her mother was under cultural pressure to produce a beautiful little girl, that is, one who fit the aesthetic prescriptions of a racist, patriarchal culture. To achieve this visual effect, she often tried to adorn Sara's hair with ribbons and laces. From a very early age, Sara would reject these ministrations and her mother, feeling like a failure, would resort to tears and name-calling. That this disconnection should be experienced on such a sensate level was key to understanding the relational images Sara formed about herself in relation to other women she categorized as white. She remembers being sent off to live with her grandmother, a Ukrainian immigrant, who lovingly provided the care–including hair braiding–that her biracial granddaughter required. Sadly, her grandmother died when Sara was six, and she and her mother were left to deal with each other as best they could.

Sara remembered that when she came out to her mother as lesbian, it was just one additional thing that her mother could not bear about her. Sara's relationship history with intimate partners was equally problematic. On one hand, she foreswore any intimate relationship with women of different races. In her words, "White women were totally off limits as potential partners." Sara had come to rely on a set of relational images that served as vigilant warnings that white women could never be responsive to or interested in her needs. On the other hand, she found herself in what she called a string of disastrous liaisons with women of color. Frequent eruptions of rage characterized these relationships, with Sara typically leaving abruptly in a panic of disgust and disappointment. One day, as we were talking about Sara's constricted relational possibilities, she became aware that what she had rationalized as "Afrocentricity" was in large measure her way of containing racialized anxiety, and that this anxiety countermanded her desire for intimate connection.

She had concluded from her experiences, first with her mother's withdrawal and then with her grandmother's death, that racial difference meant abandonment. She simply couldn't imagine a good ending to any story that featured cross-racial intimacy, and she developed quite a colorful repertoire of scenarios in which a racially different partner might emotionally and physically abandon her. She therefore lived in a state of emotional truncation, unable to acknowledge or represent the range of feelings, desires, and hopes that make intimacy possible. Ironically, her efforts to make intimate connections with same-race women were grounded in illusions of separation. That is, her efforts to form relationships with black women and other women of color were actually attempts to enact images and illusions she had developed about their being "not white." Neither she nor they were allowed the range of expression that could be the source of truer intimacy. Her decision to avoid the women she called white–in some ways these designations were quite arbitrary–led to suppressed desire and further constricted the possibilities for greater self-empathy and self-knowledge.

As Sara began to access and own the painful vulnerability she had felt as a child, she also began to access more positive images of herself in relationship with her mother. She remembered her mother as quite playful and full of good humor. In addition, she remembered that it was her mother who would advocate on her behalf with teachers who were impatient with her being a "late reader." Her mother's persistence in the face of bureaucratic powers had prevented her being consigned to a track for academically challenged students. Because these more positive memories had been suppressed along with the sense of unsafe vulnerability and abandonment, she could respond only with rage and derision to any expression of "weakness" by her mother or any of her partners.

It perhaps goes without saying that she was unable to tolerate those feelings of vulnerability in herself. Suppressing her own feeling-thoughts was her primary strategy of disconnection. It was only through disconnection that she could experience a temporary respite from the terror of her yearning. For Sara, the path to intimacy was a path through grief.

As she became more confident in her own relational capacity, she could surface the toxic anxiety, remember past hurts, mourn lost hopes, and move with courage to embrace the complexity of her own yearning.

There are those moments in life when the subtle variations of doubt and shame shape our responses to questions about meaning, hope, and connection.

Those are the moments Gerzon (1998) has described as, "Standing naked and shivering in our awareness of ourselves as skin-encapsulated bits of matter." We stand facing our aloneness and yearning for oneness. Some have referred to this inescapable dilemma of the human condition as existential anxiety; Gerzon uses the language of scared anxiety. In a culture that overemphasizes the skin-encapsulation, the separateness, it is to be expected that scared or existential anxiety might turn toxic. Furthermore, when skin itself becomes the basis of social valuation, it is to be expected that the anxiety–to which flesh is heir–might be met with relational distortions.

As Mirtha Quintanales (1983) wrote: "The social privileges of lighter-than-black are almost totally dependent upon denial of who we are . . . lighter-than-black skin may confer the option of being assimilated–integrated into mainstream American society. But is this really a privilege when it almost means having to be invisible, ghost-like, identity-less, community-less, alienated? The perils of passing as white are perils indeed–being and not being, merging and yet remaining utterly alone."

Whatever valence is accorded one's own skin, whether one's skin is called white or black or any of the multiple, creative variations in between, the perils of passing on skin color are perils that precipitate crises of relational confidence. To submit to a system of valuation based on skin color is to follow a path that leads to what Miller and Stiver have called "condemned isolation" (1997). That is, in response to the anxieties about purpose, possibility, and belonging, there is an experience of disconnection that leads one to question not only her capacity, but also her fitness for connection.

I had an occasion once to observe a workshop in which people from a number of ethnic groups were participating. As the group was commenting on its diversity, one woman who by most accounts was strikingly attractive, described herself as French and Danish. Everyone in the group stared somewhat incredulously at her brown skin, her full lips, and her dark wavy hair.

Finally one man said, "Is that all?" She replied tersely, "Yes." He pushed further: "Are you saying that you have no African heritage whatsoever, anywhere in your background?" She replied, "Not really, I do have some." He persisted, "Who?" She replied, "My father."

The circumstances were such that this woman, Beth, later became my client. Beth came into my practice two years after graduating from a preeminent law school, well on her way to a successful career in legal practice. She was plagued, however, by an emptiness that often left her scared, and she decided to begin therapy.

Early on in our sessions, Beth spoke frequently and lovingly of her mother, a woman of French and Danish background who had married Beth's African American father during the 1960s. Her mother's family did not approve. The couple divorced a few years after Beth was born; her mother, however, remained isolated and rejected by her own family. Beth was deeply grateful to her mother because, as she said, "She kept me."

Her sense of loving connection with her mother was tied to her sense of self as a burden. Along with memories of their fun times, of their mother-daughter outings wearing matching outfits, she also remembered her mother's isolation. She remembered the white men her mother dated, of whom two were not overjoyed to learn that blending into this family would also include blending with a brown-skinned little girl. She remembered specifically one who would take them out to dinner, and then say "teasingly," and loudly enough to be overheard: "Let's go so we can get this kid back to the orphanage." She remembered her mother's silence.

Beth herself was terribly lonely, and she was given to wildly indiscriminant sexual acting out, always with white men. Although she initially rationalized her behavior as enjoying her physicality, she was eventually able to address the ways in which she repeatedly put herself at risk. For example, in at least two relationships, she agreed with her partners that (1) theirs was a physical connection only, and that (2) she would completely respect their commitments to their "real" girlfriends. On one occasion, she consoled one boyfriend and "worried with him" when he started to doubt his girlfriend's fidelity. On another occasion, she helped her partner clean his apartment in preparation for his girlfriend's weekend visit. As a child who had grown up with a sense of her racial self as burdensome and problematic, Beth had come to see herself as unfit for connection. She had experienced herself as the cause of her mother's isolation and had thus concluded that she had no right to voice or choice in relationships.

To say the least, these multi-layered images, which formed over time, precipitated a crisis of relational confidence. Beth confided that in spite of her many and highly visible accomplishments, her sense of isolation and alienation were longstanding. Furthermore, she could never tell her mother about her pain for fear of adding to her mother's guilt. "When we're together," she said, "we focus mainly on the positive." It became clear that neither woman felt empowered in the relationship. In one sense, Beth felt that her mother was all she had–and to hold onto her sense of connection, Beth had all but canonized her for sainthood. To acknowledge the feelings of disappointment or anger that are part and parcel of any intimate relationship was to threaten their tenuous hold on connection.

In a culture that over-emphasizes skin-encapsulation, that is, a culture that prescribes separateness based on skin color alone, the intimacy between Beth and her mother was under relentless scrutiny and occasional assault. The relational images formed under these conditions led Beth to believe that intimacy could be measured by the extent to which racial difference could be ignored. She found it unthinkable that acknowledging feelings of sadness and disappointment could in fact lead to deeper, more resilient connection.

Any feeling that did not support the *appearance* of connection could not be represented in the relationship. Over time, Beth was able to make use of our relationship to practice "good enough" authenticity. She was able to use the relationship to expand her emotional range. She first had to recognize (often on a physical level) and then to name a fuller spectrum of emotionality. For example, she became increasingly more able to name the irritations she experienced in the therapy with me. One of Beth's strategies of disconnection in relationship with me was to offer effusive praise. As we paid attention to her care-taking efforts both by appreciating her capacity for caring and by naming her expectations for return, Beth became aware of her efforts to use praise to secure her place in a relationship. Along with voicing her awareness she was better able to examine the conclusions that defined her images of herself in relationship. Through our relationship, Beth learned to transform her feelings of anxiety into the energy of awareness; thereby increasing her confidence that she could participate in other relationships in life-enhancing ways.

One opportunity came during a signal moment in Beth's relationship with a new boyfriend, Doug, whom she liked to describe as Irish-Italian. Unlike her earlier partners, this young man viewed himself as socially progressive and seemed to enjoy engaging Beth in conversations about politics and the many "ism's" in the culture. They could actually talk about race. For the first time, Beth was in a relationship in which she felt safe to more fully represent herself. In fact, it soon became clear that both she and her partner were quite enjoying the politics of their romance. Being an interracial couple carried a certain cachet that neither had experienced before.

There they were, in defiance of and in opposition to a culture that was clearly not as progressive as they: until one evening when Beth's partner wanted to go in to a bar in which she felt very uncomfortable. Beth described the bar as having kind of a "neighborhood chumminess" filled with mostly men and a few women who had obviously been in there for the "long haul." Had they gone in, she would have been the only person of color in the bar. When she expressed her apprehension, her boyfriend initially tried to cajole her out of her concerns. When she persisted, he became somewhat strident, criticizing her for being "too insular." They agreed to go to another place, but sat in stony silence for several minutes. The night had been ruined.

Then gathering all of her courage, Beth told him, "I am feeling really scared. For the first time, I'm getting the sense that my blackness could inconvenience you, and you could resent me." Doug was stunned. Like Beth, he too had formed relational images about the meaning of racial difference. He was quite vested in his image of himself as progressive, a social iconoclast untouched by the ignorance and arrogance of racism. To enter into this conflict with Beth, to give credence to her experience was to deepen a process of mutuality never before attempted. To engage in mutual empathy required him to relinquish his hold on his image of himself. But he did; he spoke about the fear of constriction, and the loss of social acceptance he could experience as a partner in an interracial relationship. According to Beth, he was able to speak–painfully at first, but frankly–about his feelings of superiority, however fleeting, and his frustration when she spoke out of a reality that was different from his. Beth admitted the embarrassment and rage she felt at times knowing that some people viewed their relationship with skepticism or derision.

She confessed that sometimes she was afraid that people would think they were together because she was a prostitute. Sometimes she went to great pains to display the seriousness of their relationship to convince others (and I think also herself), that she was not just a playmate to be later set aside, or more poignantly–the kid who would be delivered back to the orphanage. Together, Beth and Doug created the courage to bear the previously unspeakable anxieties that threatened to pull them apart. Failure to do so would have left them with what Judy Jordan has described as a "dead zone," where old resentments smolder and creative energies lie buried. Beth and Doug were able to face their anxieties, wage good conflict, and allow for the emergence of something new.

CONCLUSION

These vignettes allow us to glimpse the complexity that these three biracial women were compelled to engage in their quest for truer, deeper connection. Lauren learned over time that the path to healing was the path of awareness. She learned to practice attunement to and representation of the rich subtleties of her own feeling-thoughts as she navigated the culture: a culture that was nonetheless stratified for all of its ambiguity. For Sara, the task was to *disinter* and *disable* the toxic anxiety that mocked her yearning for connection. Faced with the decision about whether to spend their evening in a bar, to go or not to go was never the real question for Beth and Doug. Instead the quandary was how to relinquish the comfort of relational images–images of themselves and the larger culture–that had provided them with a sense of safety, but had prevented them from achieving true intimacy.

It is important to recognize that these three courageous biracial women, however they might have described themselves (Lauren as black, half-black, Sara as Afro-centric black, and Beth as French Danish), lived in a culture that ranked their worth and desirability according to the measure of their blackness. Though it is recognized as scientifically specious, the "one drop rule" carries real consequences in a racially stratified culture. Under conditions of stratification, racial anxieties exploit the normal and inevitable conflicts that might otherwise lead to resilience and healing. It should also be said that though the dilemmas of three women are used to illustrate three types or levels of anxiety, racial anxieties are never really present in neatly compartmentalized and easily recognized form. Instead, they may be sinuously layered around everyday experience. And there is no hiding place. As the lives of three women illustrate, neither family kinship nor sexual intimacy can offer refuge from racial anxiety–which almost always erupts unbidden. In fact, to declare oneself immune by virtue of biological ties or sexual practice is to forego opportunities to deepen and enliven connection.

A first step toward relational healing is to acknowledge that we are all in and we are of it. A developmental legacy of a racially stratified culture is that its members (on both sides of the inequality) are socialized to adopt strategies of disconnection as survival skills. Failure to acknowledge that reality is to ignore, and thereby fortify, the potency of the culture as an agent of disconnection. The path to relational healing leads us on a journey fraught with risk and imbued with promise. It is a journey of courage and faith: the courage to be mindful and to grieve, to risk letting go of old relational images that function to *contain* our anxieties, in hopes of discovering and enlarging our capacity for richer authenticity. The path to relational healing invites us to enter into conflict with faith in our human possibilities and with desire for the emergence of something new.

REFERENCES

Brodkin, K. (1998). *How the Jews became white folk and what that says about race in America.* New Brunswick, NJ: Rutgers University Press.

Gerzon, R. (1998). *Finding serenity in the age of anxiety.* New York: Bantam Books.

Lorde, A. (1984). *Sister outsider: Essays and speeches.* Trumansburg, NY: Crossing Press.

Miller, J. B. (1988). Connections, disconnections, and violations. *Work in Progress, No. 33.* Wellesley, MA: Stone Center Working Paper Series.

Miller, J. B. (1986). *Toward a new psychology of women.* Boston: Beacon Press.

Miller, J. B. & Stiver, I. P. (1997). *The healing connection: How women form relationships in therapy and in life.* Boston: Beacon Press.

Quintanales, M. (1983). I paid very hard for my immigrant ignorance. In C. Moraga & G. Anzaldua (Eds.). *This bridge called my back: Writings by radical women of color.* New York: Kitchen Table, Women of Color Press.

How Therapy Helps When the Culture Hurts

Maureen Walker

SUMMARY. The purpose of psychotherapy is movement toward relational healing. However, the practice itself is embedded in a culture where relational disconnection and power-over arrangements are normative. The purpose of this article is to examine the impact of cultural disconnections on the therapy relationship. Because they embody multiple social identities within a power-over paradigm, both client and therapist are "carriers" of cultural disconnections. The article examines the shifting vulnerabilities associated with those identities that may lead to impasse and violation or contribute to possibilities for growth. Scenarios from clinical practice illustrate how conflict becomes a pathway to deeper connection when embraced with such processes as empathic attunement, authentic responsiveness, and mutuality.

Maureen Walker, PhD, is Director of Program Development, JBMTI; Associate Director of Support Services, Harvard Business School; in private practice for psychotherapy and multicultural consultation, Cambridge, MA; and co-editor of *How Connections Heal* and *The Complexity of Connection*.

This article was originally presented at the 2002 Summer Advanced Training Institute sponsored by the Jean Baker Training Institute at Wellesley College.

INTRODUCTION

It is impossible to think about movement and healing in the therapy relationship without considering the culture in which the relationship is embedded. To begin engaging the question of how therapy helps when the culture hurts, I will recount a conversation with a dear friend and colleague of mine whom I will call Claire.

Not too many years ago, Claire and I strolled the sidewalks of Santa Fe talking about where our careers had taken us since our days in graduate school together. She had recently become installed as director of a small university counseling service in the Southwest, and I was on the counseling staff of a large professional school in the East. However different our respective venues, we agreed that we had both traveled some distance from the days of videotaped supervisions and mandatory process groups–certainly memorable if not endearing parts of our graduate school experience. As somewhat newly minted therapists are prone to do, we were discussing some of our more frustrating cases, and were once again enjoying the comfort and familiarity of informal supervision together.

Claire, who is a white woman, told me about her work with another white woman, a young student who had come to the counseling center in acute distress after a break up with a boyfriend. During the course of their short time together, Claire learned that woman had a long history of abuse at the hands of men and boys. Again as newly minted *feminist* therapists are wont to do, Claire had elaborate visions of journeying with this woman on the path to empowerment, when one day the woman came into session and abruptly announced that she planned to leave the therapy. She said to Claire, "I have strong suspicions that you are a lesbian. And I don't think it would be good to work with someone like you."

I am not at all certain about the content of the conversation that followed, but I am certain of its nature. No doubt we commiserated grandly about living in a culture rife with destructive disconnections: a heterosexist culture that at its best colludes with the willful ignorance that often underlies homophobia, and at its worst rewards outright violence against lesbian, gay, transgendered, and bisexual people.

It is important to note that my friend Claire would often describe herself as bisexual–as someone who was "mostly out with some people most of the time." No doubt as she told her story, we were both self-righteously indignant: I as her straight sister-colleague who not only grieved my friend's pain, but also as a straight friend who needed to bolster my credentials as an ally. Claire, for her part was strongly identified with feminist politics and had more than a passing interest in interrupting everyday gay oppression. It is probably the case that our conversation eventually wound its way into musings on authenticity–what should Claire or any politically enlightened therapist do? Cloaked as we were in our images of ourselves and of each other, I am certain we had a comforting and familiar conversation. I am not at all certain that we had a conversation that allowed us to grow and deepen our connection with each other.

WHAT SHOULD THE THERAPIST DO?

Under the usual terms of therapeutic engagement, the question that emerges most immediately is all too often framed in binary terms: Should Claire disclose or not disclose? All too often the apparent, binary options have the potential for disempowering the relationship, where the *therapist,* the *client,* or sometimes *both* can be left in shame and isolation. From the standpoint of the Relational-Cultural Model, the question is not so much to disclose or not to disclose; the question is rather what are the makings of authenticity in this relationship?

A foundational premise for considering such a question is put forth by Elaine Pinderhughes (1989) who states that knowing how power and powerlessness operate in human systems is key to effective interventions. Inasmuch as the therapy relationship is a human system, the participants in that system must necessarily concern themselves with issues of power. It follows then that in relational-cultural practice, issues of authenticity must be understood in light of the operative power issues in the relationship. Therapists who find themselves in situations similar to Claire's can almost always craft a "good enough" response, sometimes even a true enough response. However, from the standpoint of relational-cultural practice, the *why* and *how* of our responses is almost always at least as important as the *what*. Attending to the how and the why helps us to more honestly navigate the complexities of power in the relational system.

It could be said that Claire's young client invited her into conflict with a challenge that was at once a strategy of disconnection and an invitation into deeper knowing and connection. It was a challenge that could lead to either impasse or possibility. Embedded as it was in a culture of chronic disconnection, it was a challenge that illuminated the multilayered complexities of power and powerlessness in their relationship. It is a fundamental premise of the Relational-Cultural Model that acute disconnection can lead to a deepening of connection. In other words, we learn to see acute conflict as the source of growth and possibility. Chronic disconnection on the other hand can lead to isolation, stagnation, and hopelessness. It is against this backdrop of chronic and compound disconnection that we seek to understand how therapy can help when the culture hurts.

CONFLICT AND THE "POWER-OVER" CULTURE

Every relationship, including the therapy relationship, bears the complexity of multiple social identities. That is, the bodies that we bring into relationship with each other have been formed by multiple sociocultural agendas: we have been raced, engendered, sexualized, and situated along dimensions of class, physical ability, religion, or whatever constructions carry ontological significance in the culture. In a culture of chronic disconnection, manifest difference mutates into what Jean Baker Miller (1986) calls "power-over," a cultural arrangement in which difference is stratified into dominant and subordinate, superior and inferior. In these power-over arrangements, the dominant group protects its status and perpetuates its presumed entitlements through tactics ranging from obfuscation and exclusion to violence and extermination. In addition to bearing the culturally ascribed power of each identity, our experience in relationship is made more complex by the specific images and meanings formed over time, relational images that attempt to predict and explain the meanings of and possibilities for relationship. The way we respond to the inevitable disconnections in relationship is in large measure a function of the multiple social identities operating in that particular relationship and in the relational surround at any given moment.

When Miller (1986) wrote *Toward a New Psychology of Women*, she observed that growth requires engagement with difference *and* with people *embodying* that difference. Construed simply as engagement with difference, conflict is both inevitable and necessary for growth. However in a power-over paradigm, open engagement with difference is made problematic, as the dominant group moves expeditiously and often unconsciously to suppress conflict. The therapy relationship itself is in no way immune to machinations of a power-over paradigm.

An example that I often use comes straight from my own experience in clinical supervision. I was trained in a very traditional model and on more than a few occasions I can remember various supervisors (who were no doubt trying to save us from ourselves or from our clients) admonishing us to maintain the therapeutic framework and warning us about the perils that would most certainly follow should we ever leak our power by loosening the frame. Those very same well-intentioned supervisors would also warn us to never, ever engage in power struggles with our clients. The message that I learned was this:

1. My client and I are in a contest.
2. My job as the therapist is to win it.
3. A good therapist is one who can win by pretending not to be in a contest with her client.

I exaggerate only slightly. My point is that all too often we are steeped, by tradition, in a power-over paradigm of therapy. The rules of engagement require that the therapist at all times assert her dominance in relationship and maintain power-over in relationship, lest she be overpowered. Furthermore, as in other power-over systems, she must mystify and or otherwise obscure the truth of what she is doing. It is important that we recognize the extent to which the therapy relationship is a microcosm of power and may, in fact, replicate the systems and arrangements we see in the larger world. It is also important that we recognize that both the therapist and the client are carriers of disconnection, importing into the relationship the images and strategies that perpetuate distorted power practice.

As we all know, there are multilayered power differentials operating in any given therapy relationship. There are certain inequalities that may well be, as Miller has observed, natural and essential. In the case of Claire and her client, there were differentials along dimensions of professional status (therapist and client). There is in that differential a presumption of competence and expertise that the therapist must exercise in the service of productive movement. Moreover, in relational-cultural practice the relationship functions to reduce the differential. On the other hand, power differentials that reflect stratified social identities (e.g., bisexual and straight) function in support of cultural privilege and false entitlement or systematic disadvantage and marginalization. These culturally inbred inequalities result in conflict. To ignore or suppress the conflict is to collude with the social practices that cement power differentials in place.

CONFLICT AS A SOURCE OF GROWTH

Not all conflict is the result of power-over social arrangements. Conflict is inevitable wherever people allow themselves to be known–wherever people risk deeper and fuller representation of themselves in relationship. Because therapy by design moves the participants toward greater clarity and authenticity in their relationship, it "invites" conflict as a pathway to healing and transformation. In other words, the therapy relationship is a very vulnerable place. Though not in equal measure and not at all times, the relationship is a place where client and therapist share in shifting vulnerabilities as they move toward deeper connection.

The compelling issue is how to navigate those shifting vulnerabilities in a power-over culture, where difference equals disconnection. In a power-over culture, the healing potential of conflict is easily undermined. Against such a backdrop, culturally stratified difference becomes opportunistic, exploiting the inevitable and potentially growth-producing conflicts between therapist and client. An example of this dynamic may be seen in the case of Claire and her client. Were it not for the distorted power associated with their presumed difference in sexual orientation, Claire might have viewed her client's behavior as a well-honed strategy of disconnection by a young woman probably unfamiliar with and terrified of intimacy. Interestingly, between Claire and her client lay many sources of difference. Likewise, there are multiple explanatory frameworks that can be usefully deployed to shed light on the disconnection between the two women. However, the salient difference tends to be the one where the cultural pain is, where opportunistic power is practiced. And the salient difference becomes the default explanation for the disconnection.

More likely than not, the young woman's homophobia, her cultural pain, turned opportunistic and exploited her terror of and yearning for intimacy. It is also likely that the acute conflict with her therapist served to reinforce the young woman's homophobia.

Armed with the distorted images and practices of the power-over culture, she targeted Claire's cultural pain, her ambivalence about her identifications as a sexual being. Years of anger, hurt, and shame, that Claire had held mostly in isolation for so-called safekeeping, were called into the relationship. Claire felt diminished and humiliated in her client's sight. She lacked empathic resonance with her own struggle as a bisexual woman in a world where heterosexual privilege defines the norm. She lived in fear of being "outed" against her will and experienced absolute fatigue at the ongoing-ness of her struggle.

In hindsight, our sidewalk conversation did little to shift the images that forced Claire's shame out of relationship and into isolation. It served mostly to reapportion the vulnerability, to restore Claire to her presumptive place of power in the therapy relationship. If we were to be truthful (and we mostly were not) the subtext of our indignation was "how dare this needy, hapless client *presume* to assert her superiority over the wise and mostly beneficent therapist?" The fact is that we were collusive with a paradigm that would cast the client as the sole carrier of the vulnerability in therapy relationship.

We also remained oblivious to ways in which both the client and the therapist are carriers of cultural disconnection. The irony is that by accepting the usual terms of engagement, we in no way challenged the power-over paradigm that oppressed both client and therapist, casting them in roles not just *different* from each other, but in *opposition to* each other: healthy or sick, victim or oppressor, powerful or vulnerable.

FALLACIES OF A BINARY PARADIGM

Irene Stiver often commented that real impasse in therapy occurs when the therapist disconnects in *reaction* to the client's disconnection. There are few more potent strategies of disconnection than enshrouding oneself in the mantle of "victim-ness." Let me be very clear: there is no way to overstate the effects of abusive power, whether it is emotional, physical, sexual, or cultural. Abusive power creates real victims and one way out of that victimization is to begin naming it, to begin the process of representing the fullness and complexity of the pain. A unidimensional representation of cultural pain serves primarily to solidify the relational images that create binary categories of victim or oppressor. Furthermore, a unidimensional representation of conflict creates a binary frame where the victim may not only absolve herself of relational accountability but also rob herself of the complex potentialities of her own "feelingthoughts." A unidimensional representation of cultural pain reproduces the functions of a binary, power-over framework.

In the initial sharing of the story, Claire is cast as the therapist victimized by an ungrateful, woefully or willfully ignorant client. For the client to assert her greater social power (i.e., heterosexual privilege) over her bisexual therapist was an act of profound ingratitude. By doing so, the young woman upended our image of proper relationship between therapist and client. After all, if giving support is the prerogative of the powerful (read: therapist), then expressing gratitude is the obligation of the powerless (read: client). The client's refusal to remain in her proper place in the paradigm of power-over therapy represented not just personal affront, but also an assault on the relational expectations fed by the controlling images of the Good Therapist (i.e., unfailingly wise, confident, and available). Given that both client and therapist bring the chronic disconnection of the culture into the therapy relationship, an almost default reaction to a disconnection is to move swiftly to repair the images that offer the illusion of protection and invulnerability. However, movement toward the images is movement out of the relationship. When our experience of disconnection propels us toward the illusory protection of relational or controlling images, the result is often stagnating conflict.

Sadly, we all are witness to devastating violations that occur when conflict in the world and interpersonal arenas is defined by a reactive paradigm of power-over, where the possible courses of response are derived from the standpoint of dichotomy: victim or oppressor, powerful or vulnerable, righteous or evil.

One of the consequences of such binary framing of disconnection is loss of relational accountability. From the standpoint of unidimensional victim-hood, one is justified, even wise to enact any strategy necessary to regain the illusion of control, or at the very minimum to stave off any possibility of threat. At this point in our national consciousness, we are all too familiar with the expressions and repercussions of binary thinking. We may be less familiar with the manifestations in the interpersonal, or more specifically, the therapeutic arena. As clinicians, what we sometimes call interventions are well-disguised strategies of disconnection and control. Sometimes they may take the form of a too swift retort–otherwise called confrontation–that serves little purpose other than alleviating the therapist's anxiety, or more punitively, reducing the client back to a manageable size. For example, when a client gets "out of place" by asking a question that makes the therapist feel inadequate, anxious, or otherwise out of control, the therapist may react by shaming him or her for asking the question: she can easily generate some response that suggests the client is too sick to know the answer, or that her asking is the sign of some pathology. Whatever form such an intervention takes, too often the unspoken intent is to restore the apportionment of power.

Another consequence of binary framing of power is what I call *exclusionary entrapment*. That is, we become over-identified with particular images of self or relationship: images that valorize one part of our experience to the exclusion or denigration of other parts of our experience. For example, if I as a therapist am committed to and sustained by an image of myself as ever-available, patient, and wise, I am less likely to be empathically attuned to any experiences that contradict that image of myself. I am less likely to be patient with or aware of my shame about my own imperfections, my capacity for disconnection and harm to another. Again, Claire's situation with her client serves to illustrate this point. Attached as she was to the image of herself as a savvy feminist therapist wholly committed to the empowerment of all women, she was less empathic with what she experienced as weakness and vulnerability in herself. She was therefore unable to represent the fullness and complexity of her experience to herself or to others.

Images that are maintained through isolation from actual relationship function to entrap. They constrain our explanatory options: we have difficulty making sense of or understanding the why of our experience. They limit our sense of possibility; we become reactive and have difficulty discerning what is good for the relationship in the moment. To the extent that Claire was entrapped in isolation with her images of the Ideal Therapist and the Good Client, she was unable to risk the empathic attunement and relational authenticity that would allow her to grow in relationship with her client.

HOW AUTHENTIC RESPONSIVENESS PROMOTES MOVEMENT TOWARD HEALING

In order for healing conflict to emerge, authenticity is required. The therapist needs to allow herself to be known. It is important to say here that authenticity is not the same as reactive disclosure. Judy Jordan (personal communication, April 2002) makes a very useful distinction between responsiveness, that is attunement to the relationship and reactivity. Reactivity is not authenticity. In fact, it may well function to entrap. Instead of promoting movement and clarity, it may in fact perpetuate the status quo. Authenticity heals cultural pain when there is a commitment to empathic attunement, and relational accountability. Accordingly, how the therapist deals with the shame and anger of her own cultural pain determines the quality of authenticity. It is authentic responsiveness, empathic attunement, and accountability to the relationship that allows healing conflict to emerge.

Authentic responsiveness to the relationship facilitates awareness of the multiple social identities and the multiple systems of meaning operating in the relationship. More often than not, we turn our attention to those identities that are socially problematized, while the problematic aspects of socially privileged identities remain all but invisible. Great power resides in privileged invisibility. Protected by its invisibility, the dominant group can impose its own story on relationship, set the definitional frames and terms of engagement with little to no accountability.

I recall a few years ago I was doing a consultation with a group of middle managers representing various industries. One of the managers contended that in her organization there were no problems with race, because as she put it: "There are no black people. We are all the same." This kind of thinking is perhaps more prevalent than one might hope or imagine, and it speaks to a very dangerous split in our national consciousness.

Janet Helms (1992) has spoken eloquently and often about the dangers of defining one's being wholly in opposition to one's image of another. She goes on to say that whether one is located on the dominant or the subjugated side of the inequality one cannot talk about models of personality without examining the impact of racial socialization in this culture. To talk about personality without addressing racial socialization is to participate in the evolution of what some cultural anthropologists call the binary self–a self formed in opposition to images of the Degraded Other. Because it is shaped by anxious reactivity to images rather than through meaningful participation in relationship, this type of self-construction may be experienced as profound emptiness (Cushman, 1997).

If we are to move toward healing the wounds of cultural disconnection, it is important that we problematize the assumptive frameworks of dominance in our clinical practice. The silent and invisible assumptions determine what we see and what we fail to see, what we scrutinize and what we fail to examine. For example, it is not at all unusual for clinicians to engage in discussions about the impact of race or sexuality on people with socially degraded status. Far less time is devoted to speculating about the impact of socially privileged status on mental health. It is as if we are saying in our research *and* in our clinical practices, that socially privileged status is non-problematic. For example, for more than a few years, studies were conducted associating homosexuality with depression, and female gender with particular personality disorders. Similarly, in graduate training programs, conversations often took place about the causes and meanings of abbreviated treatment when black clients have white therapists. We find far fewer studies examining the causes and meaning of abbreviated treatment when white clients have black therapists or the impact of race when white clients are choosing therapists. We see far fewer investigations asking if there is a link between heterosexuality and anxiety or male gender and certain personality disorders.

I am not advocating that we should. I *am* suggesting that the questions we ask, what we see or fail to see is a telling indicator of the implicit operation of power in our cultural system. When we fail to interrogate the assumptive frameworks of social privilege, the dominant culture by default will impose its own story and disallow the multilayered narratives operating in the therapy relationship.

It is interesting to note that certain models of therapy *require* that the therapist remain all but invisible. It is important to recognize that invisibility can support power-over and from such a paradigm certain questions and possibilities will never surface.

Authentic responsiveness in relationship allows the therapist and client to interrogate the assumptive frameworks of dominance that constrain clarity and possibility. When the assumptions go unchallenged there exists a heightened risk that participants in a relationship will construct relational images patterned along the lines of the controlling images of the culture. They seek to fit their stories into the binary patterns that the culture provides, stripping themselves of texture, complexity, dignity, and possibility.

To illustrate let me offer again the case of Claire and her client. Sometime during their work together, Claire learned that in her young client's long history of abuse, all of her romantic involvements had been with men of color. Although initially repelled by what she saw as her client's paradoxical mixture of arrogance and naiveté, Claire used the opportunity–as one white woman to another–to talk about the meaning of race and gender in this woman's life. Claire learned that when her client was a young girl, she was molested by her older brother. Having internalized the premises of white supremacy and gender subordination, she then determined that no other white man would ever want her–that in fact, she was not pretty enough or good enough for a white boyfriend. The painful irony of her situation is that she sought safety–and called it intimacy–in relationship with people to whom she felt superior. Through a multiplicity of controlling images, the assumptive framework of dominance renders dichotomous options: the Idealized and the Despised. Both result in shame. Having failed in measuring up to her image of the Idealized White Woman, Claire's client saw herself as the embodiment of the Despised. Again, we can see how the controlling images promoted by the dominant culture provided the broad outlines of her story: the client herself connected the dots with relational images that cast her as unworthy of connection, except with persons more unworthy than herself.

In many ways, this young woman embodied the emptiness of the binary self. In fact, what we see as cultural arrogance or its binary opposite, loathing, is often an expression of profound emptiness, and it creates pockets of isolation in relationship. That which cannot be represented in relationship remains under the silencing control of the dominant images. In other words these images can render both the therapist and the client voiceless. By interrogating the silent assumptions and controlling images of whiteness, Claire was beginning to help her client *transform* her shame and recognize her capacity for shaming others. She was beginning to recognize her own voice and to grow in her capacity for resonance *with* her own desires.

HOW MUTUALITY PROMOTES MOVEMENT TOWARD HEALING

Chronic cultural disconnection eviscerates desire. To risk desire is to risk awareness of uncertainty and openness to possibility. In a culture that valorizes power-over as the means to physical survival, emotional safety, and material well-being, openness and uncertainty are dangerous options indeed. Therefore, when we enter into a therapeutic relationship with the goal of increasing capacity for relational responsiveness, we are engaging a counter-cultural process. We are engaging the process of transforming *generations-old* shame and anger, intensified by inevitable, *everyday* disconnections of the power-over culture. Irrespective of the seeming similarities or differences between client and therapist, the therapy relationship is both juxtaposed against and reflective of this milieu of disconnection. It was in this milieu of disconnection that I found myself in a relationship with a client whom I will call Brad.

At the time of this focal incident, Brad and I had been working together for almost two years. Brad was a 47-year-old African American who had moved to the Boston area from the West Coast to work in the computer software industry. Brad was a gay man. Often in therapy, Brad spoke of his unrelenting loneliness and his difficulty finding a partner willing to be in an open, committed relationship. He also attributed much of this difficulty to geography and almost weekly lamented the fact that Boston is such a "white world." And in spite of his loneliness, on an almost weekly basis, Brad would vow that *never* would he consider taking a white lover. Somewhat in response to his assertions, we had a few conversations about his experience of race and the intersecting oppressions of race and sexuality–in some respects, well-rehearsed conversations on both our parts that did little to increase the learning in our relationship. Not surprisingly, these conversations did little to move him any closer to resolving his dilemma. Once when Brad reported a particularly problematic work situation, we began discussing the availability of mentors or allies. It turned out that Brad's immediate supervisor was an African American male, with whom he had a pleasant and respectful relationship. However, Brad continued, "I could never really trust him with anything real. After all, he's married to a white woman."

It occurred to me to wonder if Brad knew that I, myself, was in an interracial marriage, married to a white man. As in the situation with Claire and her client, the obvious, immediate question was framed in binary terms: to disclose or not to disclose? Like Claire and her client, we were both carriers of cultural disconnection. Whatever Brad knew or did not know, the truth of the moment was that we faced each other, both carriers of generations-old shame and anger, fortified by decades-old relational images. We faced each other as carriers of images formed under the interlocking constraints of racism, sexism, and heterosexism in our culture.

SO WHAT SHOULD THE THERAPIST DO?

Again, the apparent question is not always the compelling question. The compelling question before us was not about disclosure or nondisclosure, but rather how to gain the clarity and courage to embrace a potentially healing and empowering conflict. It was helpful for me to pause long enough to connect with the feelings-thoughts that emerged and morphed as we continued the conversation. It is usually during these moments of noticing that I can connect with the support and holding I have received from supervisors and mentors over the years: people like Irene Stiver who always reminded us that in moments of confusion or complexity, we can usually find one true thing to say that will (1) keep us connected to the relationship and (2) allow other truths to emerge. I recall that in the moment my "true thing" was to make some comment about how difficult it is to be open, even to "growth opportunities" when one feels so fundamentally unsafe. Perhaps later we talked more about his wariness around black people whom he saw as "sellouts." As the conversation went on, Brad acknowledged that his criteria for judging someone as a sellout could be as diverse as how the person chooses a mate to their aesthetic taste in home furnishings. Also, Brad began to remember what he called his own self-loathing, as he had to contend in his formative years with both gay oppression and racial oppression. When the hour was up we took our leave, but in no way was the session over.

As my feelings emerged and shifted, I continued to consider the meaning of authenticity in our relationship, as well as how the process of mutuality would unfold. It was very clear to me that any so-called disclosure could serve just as much to silence Brad as to signal respect. Likewise any interpretations about projections and such, while possibly true, seemed more like battle strategies to preserve my power in my professional territory. (Old controlling images of the good therapist: Never let your client put you on the hot seat–they'll do whatever they can to take the focus off themselves.) It was as important to consider the impact of our seeming similarities, as it was our apparent differences. Brad and I identified with a racially subjugated group: both of us are African Americans, both born in roughly the same generation of our nation's history. We share a silent knowledge born of that shared history. The poet Carolyn Rodgers (1975) spoke of this silent knowledge when she wrote:

> All the people I know I know too well. There is comfort in that sometimes, but it also means we know each other's miseries too well.

Our shared history meant that Brad and I knew each other's miseries quite well, and often that *knowing* was a source of shame and disconnection. For example, we both knew the history of the sexual servitude of black women to white men. We both know the ways in which race and sex are implicated in the subjugation, division, destruction–the disconnections between black women and men in this country. Being authentic in relationship with Brad required that I once again examine my life and reconnect (become empathic with) both my ancient shame and actual desire in light of that history. It also meant noticing how that shared history affected my ability to be open to Brad's perceptions in our conflict. What indeed is the meaning of mutuality in this instance? What did it mean to sit eyes to eyes–seeing clearly and knowing that what we saw could transform us both?

It was becoming increasingly clear that my task in our evolving relationship was to soften my "boundedness" to make room for Brad's impact and to be available to his perceptions of and feelings about our shared history. For instance, he talked about his anger–actually his contempt–for African Americans who attempt to become racially invisible in order to avoid seeing history. We also talked about the paradox of hyper-visibility as a strategy of disconnection: a subterfuge to avoid facing the personal ravages of intergenerational shame and ambivalence. As we sat face-to-face, eyes-to-eyes, it became increasingly clear that mutuality depended upon acknowledging the incipient wisdom of his wariness. It also meant co-creating a space of transformational possibility: where Brad could bear seeing how the images that he thought would *protect* him from his past history and his present vulnerability were also images that trapped him in anger and isolation.

In order to approach the possibility of mutually empowering conflict, I was also compelled to pay attention to the operative power differentials in our relationship. Clearly and most poignantly for him, I was the face of heterosexual privilege. I enjoyed a certain amount of cultural privilege, or whatever social capital one receives from living in a committed, heterosexual relationship. I carried professional privilege; I was after all the therapist in the room and could well have exercised that power in a way that left him feeling shamed and minimized. I could imagine that had I reacted to his comment by revealing that I too was married to a white person–under the guise of therapeutic confrontation–in the moment, Brad might have felt profoundly embarrassed. Our relationship did not need that shame. Likewise, it felt a bit too self-serving to use my professional privilege to decide that sharing personal information was not good for Brad. (While that might have in fact been true, it might just as well have been a strategy for managing my own anxiety.) Although Brad was not focused on it at the time, I was aware of his gender privilege, as I noticed once again my own inclination both to shrink under the disapproving gaze of an older brother *and* to rage against the presumptuousness of his judgments. Here again, the cultural pain is opportunistic, exploiting the images, hurts, or unresolved ambivalence of our developmental histories.

In preparation for this talk, Brad and I have reviewed this episode and interestingly, neither of us recalls the exact timing or circumstances in which my own interracial marriage was discussed. We both know that weeks, perhaps months, passed. We also recalled that when it was discussed, some part of the conversation was about living in the complexity of cultural pain and personal intimacy.

I asked Brad if he recalled how he felt about the intervening weeks of nondisclosure: specifically, if he felt manipulated in light of the eventual disclosure. Brad responded that during the intervening weeks (1) my marriage was *not* uppermost on his mind; (2) our time together in the intervening weeks was allowing him to examine the racial images that constrained his movement in the world; (3) that in our talks he was forced to examine his own history of a string of unfortunate liaisons with same race men in which he had been both victim and victimizer, thus concluding that there was no safety in images. And fourth, he said that when I mentioned something one day about Maine and lobsters, he knew that some white people must be involved. He had also concluded in light of *our* actual relationship that eating lobsters in Maine (presumably with white people) didn't make me a "race traitor." For my part, I shared with Brad the importance of my sitting with the voices of ambivalence, shame, and anger in our relationship knowing that somehow we both had brought them in. I also shared that it was important to me as a therapist to remain empathic with those voices, believing that they could lead our relationship to new levels of empowerment and resilience.

FROM CONFLICT THROUGH GRIEF TO CONNECTION

In their last major work together, Jean Baker Miller and Irene Stiver (1997) signaled the importance of honoring the strategies of disconnection that the client brings into therapy, with the understanding that those strategies represent both a yearning for and a terror of connection. I think we can also say that strategies of disconnection signal the emergence of potentially healing conflict, and to suppress those strategies is to risk losing transformational possibility. In other words, the conflict opens a pathway flowing through grief to connection.

Over the years, my husband and I have had the opportunity to work with communities of people who are committed to anti-racism as a spiritual journey. One of the metaphors we often use to describe cross-racial connection is that of a being in a boat that leaves safe harbor to get to another shore. In the midst of the journey we find ourselves at sea encountering raging storms: storms of anger, guilt, humiliation, and sometimes despair. One of his favorite sayings is that if you don't encounter the storm, perhaps you're not in the boat. Perhaps you've found a way to stay safely on the shore. We are cultural beings, and thereby carriers of the wounds of chronic, multi-layered, and intersecting disconnection. If in our relationships we do not encounter the wounds, perhaps we are not in the boat. Perhaps the extent to which we avoid conflict is the extent to which we avoid connection. And, if our only model of conflict is that which destroys, humiliates, suppresses, or otherwise overpowers, it would make sense that we would avoid the hard work of transforming disconnection. And unfortunately, what we are all too often left with is the mere *illusion* of connection.

I believe it is Stephen Levine (2000) who suggests that unwillingness to investigate our disconnections keeps us from experiencing true connection: that fear of our own hostilities, resentments, and imperfections keeps us from knowing profound love.

In these very troubled times, I am so often reminded of the words of Irene Stiver, who was unwavering in her belief that the work of therapy is a work of faith. It is a work of faith to allow healing conflict to emerge in relationship. It is a work of faith to accept that empathy is more than just a nice word. It's risky business to sit face to face and see through another's eyes. That authenticity is more than mere honesty. It's the hard and often frightening work of making a commitment to attunement and accountability. That mutuality is more than sharing power or compromise (though that may occasionally be the appropriate thing to do). Mutuality is the willingness to embrace vulnerability–to release old defining images that promise boundaries of protection, in favor of opening oneself to the expansion and deepening that comes from growing in relationship. To paraphrase Levine (2000), it is desire–our yearning for connection that precedes anger, and underneath the anger, the conflict if you will, is an enormity of sadness–sadness at our wounded-ness. And underneath the sadness is an ocean of love.

I would like to close with an adaptation of a poem (Larkin, 1992) about journeying toward intimacy and connection across the barriers of cross-cultural pain:

> So we say to each other
> "Let us get in the boat and cross to the other side."
> Getting in the boat and making the
> "crossing" is for me, about getting close to desire.
> And I feel the terror . . .
> Alienation so clearly seen
> and even transformed.
> Love creating–so
> unexpected, so filled.
> Desire
> so deeply liberated.
> Racism has played such havoc in our lives.
> Leaving us almost dead on the shore.
> The storm of the crossing
> reveals our safety to be
> so thin,
> so quiet,
> so empty.
> Who would have ever

thought that we would meet and see
eyes to eyes.
Eyes that when we can bear to look are so filled with
longing.
They see long
Looking for a place to rest now and then
from seeing so much.
Come my sister. I have an inward
sea. A wounded-ness that does not heal.
I have been wounded by Desire,
using eyes like yours,
penetrating and creating
a life space,
a flow of water that
weeps endlessly in the freedom of yearning.
Come,
Embrace the wound
feeling
free, safe, alive.
Come, don't run away. Stay and
look into my eyes. The depth of
your brown vision reveals the darkness
that holds us
Giving birth to our
trust.
Come, my brother. Let us weep and
laugh for joy, as all the powers
of death and principalities of might
collapse and crumble
just because we dare to
see
each other
eyes to eyes.

REFERENCES

Helms, J. (1992). *A race is a nice thing to have.* Topeka, KS: Content Communications.
Larkin, W. D. (1992). *To Wed.* Unpublished poem, Natick, MA.
Levine, S., & Levine, O. (2000). *To love and be loved: The difficult yoga of relationship.* New York: Sounds True, Inc.

Miller, J. B. (1986). *Toward a new psychology of women.* Boston: Beacon Press.
Miller, J. B., & Stiver, I. P. (1997). *The healing connection.* Boston: Beacon Press.
Pinderhuges, E. (1989). *Understanding race, ethnicity, and power: The key to efficacy in clinical practice.* New York: The Free Press/Simon and Schuster.
Rodgers, C. (1975). "Poem for some black women." In *How i got ovah: New and selected poems.* Garden City, NY: Anchor Press/Doubleday.

SECTION TWO:
THE IMPORTANCE OF POWER

Introduction to Section Two: The Importance of Power

In the second section of the volume, we examine the effects of power. Jean Baker Miller's "How Change Happens: Controlling Images, Mutuality and Power" examines the inevitability of change. She extends Patricia Hill Collins's concept of controlling images and looks at the ways these images interact with relational images and strategies of disconnection to obstruct growth on both the societal and the personal levels. Maureen Walker then looks at the ways that power is associated with hyper-competitiveness and over-control. Walker examines and challenges, the "protective illusions" of the power-over paradigm. This section ends with Jean Baker Miller's last "Work in Progress, Telling the Truth about Power." This article suggests methods to help therapists acknowledge their power and suggests ways to change from power-over actions to mutually empowering relationships.

How Change Happens: Controlling Images, Mutuality, and Power

Jean Baker Miller

SUMMARY. Change is inevitable but it can go in a positive direction toward growth or in a negative direction. Extending Patricia Hill Collins' concept of controlling images (2000), we can see how these images interact with relational images and strategies of disconnection to obstruct growth on both the societal and the personal level. In therapy, change is defined as movement-in-relationship toward better connection; and increased connection leads to growth. Several aspects of therapy that lead to deeper and wider connection are explored, especially increasing the patient's power. Prior versions of parts of this article were presented at the Jean Baker Miller Summer Training Institutes in 2001 and 2002 and at the 2002 Learning from Women Conference sponsored by the Jean Baker Miller Training Institute and the Harvard Medical School/Cambridge Hospital in Boston, Massachusetts.

As therapists, we're "in the business" of change–change for the better. That's our goal. Another word for change for the better is growth. Change is the essence of life. It is most obvious in children but it is a necessity

---

Jean Baker Miller, MD (1927-2006), was Founding Scholar and Director of the Jean Baker Miller Training Institute at the Stone Center, Wellesley College; Clinical Professor of Psychiatry at Boston University School of Medicine; author of *Toward a New Psychology of Women*; and co-author of *The Healing Connection* and *Women's Growth in Connection*. She was a practicing psychiatrist and psychoanalyst.

through all of life. Change will occur inevitably but it can go in a positive or a negative direction. Further, I believe change toward growth creates pleasure. We feel most alive and zestful when we are engaged in this expanding activity.

INTRODUCTION

As therapists, we're "in the business" of change–change for the better. That's our goal. Another word for change for the better is growth. Change is the essence of life. It is most obvious in children but it is a necessity through all of life. Change will occur inevitably but it can go in a positive or a negative direction. Further, I believe change toward growth creates pleasure. We feel most alive and zestful when we are engaged in this expanding activity.

CHANGE AND RELATIONAL IMAGES

I'd like to explore the use of Relational-Cultural Theory (RCT) to further our understanding of change and its difficulties. Growthful change occurs as we encounter new experience, and this new experience usually happens in interaction with other people. We do not usually grow and develop in isolation. I think growth requires the ability to modify our relational images or to construct new ones. To do this, we must open ourselves to the influence of others. We've defined relational images (RIs) as the inner constructions we each create out of our experience in relationships (Miller & Stiver, 1997). We begin to construct them early in life, and we modify and develop them repeatedly. They define what we believe will happen to us. Not only do they portray what we expect will happen in relationships, they determine the meanings of this experience for our total conception of ourselves. For example, if our relationships have made us feel valuable, we will tend to carry this belief over to most realms of life, in school, work, or others. For the most part, we do not construct these images consciously.

To take in new experience in a growthful way, we probably compare the experience to the RIs we've created to date, again not usually consciously. If our relational images are relatively flexible, we may then modify them. However, if they have been reinforced very powerfully, and especially with threats of isolation and condemnation, we will build more rigid RIs. They will be much harder to change.

For example, a little four-year-old girl, Lucy, was very curious and gleeful. For their own reasons her parents couldn't join her in these interests and joy. She began to develop the image that when she pursued her interests no one would be there. As time went on, these RIs became rigidified into, "Whenever I pursue my interests, I will be isolated." As happens when a child feels isolated, she also developed the belief that something was "wrong" with her if she landed in this dreadful place.

Another child may be more fortunate; she may find other people, a teacher, a grandmother, or other relative who can join her in her interests and joy. She may be able to alter some of her RIs or create some new contrasting images. Perhaps she will be in conflict.

SOCIETAL CONTEXT

Therapists working with people in marginalized groups cannot think about what will help people to change without thinking about change in a larger context. For example, they can't think that things are fine for African American youth and they should just adapt to the status quo. Or that working-class youth face no obstacles but their own.

Many therapists didn't consider a need for societal change for the dominant group until they were challenged by their disciplines to become culturally competent. For others, the women's movement opened up the whole question of the norms held out for white women. This elucidation has led to questioning the norms for people of both genders and the whole construction of gender. More recently, led by marginalized women, feminists have begun to explore the intersection of race, class, and gender.

In her book, *Black Feminist Thought* (2000), Patricia Hill Collins, a sociologist and one of the scholars leading the exploration of this intersection, has suggested the concept of "controlling images." Maureen Walker referred to this idea in another paper (Walker & Miller, 2000). I find this concept provides a valuable link between the social and the psychological. Collins discusses the controlling images (CIs) inflicted on African American women. Several other authors have also discussed them, including Elizabeth Sparks in a paper on African American mothers for example, "the Mammy," "Jezebel," or, more recently, "the welfare queen" (1998).

I believe the concept can be extended to all the groups that society creates. Society also defines some groups as better than others. Working-class people can be portrayed as dimwitted, burly, uncouth, brash, and the like. White women have been described as either Madonnas or whores. In Hispanic traditions the Virgin Mary image has been very powerful.

Controlling images define who and what we each are. They determine what is acceptable and what is not, what people can do and cannot do. They exert a powerful impact on how we can act and how we construct relationships. Consequently, CIs create the framework within which people make the kinds of relationships that go into the construction of RIs. We fashion RIs in the immediate interactions in our lives. They form the psychological constructions we then carry in our minds, often without awareness. But the RIs are very determined and in many societies constricted and limited by the CIs. We are often not fully aware of the operation of CIs, although members of marginalized groups may be more conscious of them than members of the dominant group.

Collins (2000) defines all of the controlling images as lies, falsities. Although false, they exert a powerful force holding people of all groups in their place, that is, resisting change. Therefore, CIs can induce people of both privileged and non-privileged groups to believe that change cannot and should not occur. For example, white women were led to believe that they must adhere to the dominant group's image of the good heterosexual woman or they will fall to the level of "those other people," the "bad women," the "Jezebels," the "sluts," or the "dykes." They will sink into these "degraded groups."

But it is more complicated. While CIs affect us powerfully, people also create forces resisting them. These resistances may arise from two major sources. One is the truth of their own experience, which differs from these falsities. For people in marginalized groups, their group culture may reinforce these truths and convey different traditions. For example, African American people know a different story about African American women, or Latina women know that they are not docile victims. However, it can be complex for people to hold on to their truths when bombarded by the CIs.

Second, particularities within a person's immediate development may counter the CIs. For example, while a working-class family may convey to a child that s/he can't aspire too much, a parent may, in the very immediate way s/he relates to the child, convey that s/he is most precious and valuable. This attitude can form a base for the child's ability to counter restrictive images.

In sum, our society, and certainly others too, constructs groupings of people, maintains that some are better than others, forces CIs onto people, and reinforces them powerfully. It thus creates a whole framework of thinking in terms of "better than" and "less than," which is a mentality we all internalize to varying degrees. Such societies are geared to reinforcing the *status quo*. They do not build into the very workings of society a good way of learning how to "do change" well, to live in a process of change. Yet we all have to.

THREAT OF ISOLATION

What happens when we try? We have proposed that the most frightening human experience is psychological isolation (Miller, 1988). If severe, a person usually feels, along with isolation, a sense that s/he cannot be heard or understood, cannot affect the others around her–that is, she is powerless. Along with this experience is the sense that you, yourself are the reason for this. We've called this terrifying experience "condemned isolation" (Miller, 1988).

While not all threats of isolation are as horrifying as this, we all experience some degree of them. As a result, we all try to stay out of vulnerability and risk. In the attempt to do so, we create the "Central Relational Paradox" (Miller, 1988). We deeply desire and need connections but we become so afraid of what happens when we attempt to connect with the people important to us, that we keep large parts of ourselves out of connection. Those are the perceptions, thoughts, and actions that have seemed unacceptable or dangerous in the relationships surrounding us in our development. We develop what Irene Stiver called "strategies of disconnection" (SDs) (Miller & Stiver, 1997). Sometimes they are strategies for psychological survival. Again, most of this process goes on outside of our awareness.

To be open to change to new and unknown experience always potentially threatens our strategies of disconnection and our old relational images. We developed these strategies in the attempt to avoid isolation and the RIs portray our fears about the worst things that can happen in relationships. Thus, change threatens us with isolation along with powerlessness without the strategies that we believe we need and that we cling to so desperately. In sum, the big threat is isolation–and the big answer is connection. We have to keep finding the meaningful connections that will help us to encounter all of the vulnerability and risk we face in trying to change and grow. But what if we can't find the ways to become more connected? This is where therapy can come in. It is a way to help a person whose particular combination of CIs, RIs, and SDs is interfering with her ability to change.

CHANGE IN THERAPY

Overall, therapy means "movement in relationship" toward better connection. This connection will make it possible for a person to change her restrictive CIs, RIs, and SDs. But to do so, she does have to encounter "the new." In this case it is the therapist who is the bearer of new experience.

In the past, we've tried to describe some of the main processes in therapy that lead to change (Miller & Stiver, 1997). I'll summarize them briefly.

The therapist must be able to "feel with" the patient and the patient must "feel the therapist feeling with her." In saying this, we include the thoughts that go with all feelings. This is mutual empathy as it occurs in therapy.

The central guide at all times is that the therapist should be aware of how connected or disconnected she feels.

The therapist must "honor the patient's strategies of disconnection." She must recognize the powerful reasons for their existence, often born out of great pain and fear. Not only must she know this, she must be able to "feel with" the patient's deep need to cling to them.

Through this work, patient and therapist can come to understand the CIs, RIs, and SDs, how and why they come into play and feel so essential.

As a person brings more of the truth of her experience into the relationship, she finds she has become both a stronger, more developed person and also more connected to the therapist and eventually to others in her life. That is, she discovers a reversal of the *Central Relational Paradox* (Stiver, Rosen, Surrey, & Miller, 2000; for a description of the Central Relational Paradox see Miller & Stiver, 1997).

Of course, there is much more to be said about each of these points but I want to emphasize three additional possibilities. First, I believe that in addition to feeling that the therapist feels with her, a patient has to feel that change matters to the therapist and that she, the patient, matters to the therapist. It's very hard for a person to attempt all of the vulnerability and risk of trying to disrupt her CIs, RIs, and SDs if the other person is sitting there trying to act as if it doesn't matter.

I believe the relationship, and the patient, and change in the relationship do matter to the therapist. Traditionally, therapists have been encouraged not to show it or even admit it to ourselves. This differs from pressuring someone that she must change or change in the way the therapist wants or needs for her own psychological reasons. Such pressure is especially dangerous if the therapist is not aware of her own motives.

It is also different from the therapist not understanding and respecting each person's pace or, again, honoring her strategies of disconnection. It is about the therapist's real desire for the patient to reduce her suffering and distress and to grow and enlarge. It is also about the growth the therapist will inevitably experience when they both are engaged in mutually empowering movement.

This leads to the next point: change requires mutuality in movement. If growth is to occur in any relationship, both–or all–of the people involved have to change. For example, a child must change and grow; to foster that growth the rest of the family has to keep growing. They, too, learn and enlarge as they change to meet the child's growth. Sometimes this growth is easy for parents, sometimes it is much more difficult and anguishing.

In the larger society too, subordinate or marginalized groups are the ones who most need to create change but this growth usually requires that the dominant group change as well. This is the hardest part. To take a relatively easy example, if women make changes in the workplace so that they gain more flex-time, men may have to adapt to working at an altered schedule. Ultimately, the men often find that such changes benefit them, too, and benefit the whole system, as Joyce Fletcher and her colleagues elucidate in their work (Fletcher, 1999; Rapaport, Bailyn, Fletcher, & Pruitt, 2002). The whole system changes and enlarges. As we know, some systems are much more difficult to change and necessary changes are still to come as in the civil rights movement, workers' struggles, the women's movement, gay liberation, and others.

As we can see clearly in these examples, mutuality does not mean sameness or even equality. The child and the parent grow in different ways and at different rates. It is similar in therapy. The patient comes seeking change. For this change to occur, the therapist has to keep changing, for example, to meet the need for empathy with each thought and feeling as it arises, to understand and feel with each phase of the strategies of disconnection, and the like. Most of all, we need to move into those places where we feel vulnerable and at risk if the therapy calls for it. Again, this is the hardest part.

Perhaps a brief example will illustrate this notion. In doing therapy, I found it particularly difficult whenever I felt like I didn't know what to do or when I felt like I was not doing enough. I believed that I must understand *everything* about therapy and apply it appropriately. This idea was certainly reinforced by the CIs in my medical training.

With one patient, Pam, I kept feeling I was failing miserably on all of these counts. She wanted to be able to make relationships with other people and kept losing the few she made. She was a very demanding and critical person and appeared totally unaware of how she put people off. I had tried everything I could think of and we were getting nowhere. I was feeling helpless, not good enough, angry with her for making me feel this way, and then, as Maureen Walker has pointed out, ashamed of all of these feelings. Now, I was occupied with myself and, therefore, disconnected–thus, according to all of our precepts, doing the worst thing possible.

One day, after Pam complained again, I said, without really planning to, "You know I feel helpless." I was immediately very frightened. A doctor never says such a thing. More important, I believed that in most instances it is a terrible thing to say to a patient. It will make her feel utterly despairing. Thus, I was certainly moving into the unknown. I didn't know what would happen except that she would say, "That's because you're not a good therapist," and stomp out of the room. What Pam did say was, "Well, now maybe you know how I feel."

Now, I certainly felt much more involved in the next moments and so was she. She came around to saying she couldn't imagine I ever felt helpless. Here I am such an established professional. I said I often did and so did other people I knew. But I also really had faith in this process and that people working at it together can keep finding ways to move. Incidentally, her response was interesting because I had said many times, "I know it's so hard to feel so alone." I certainly meant it. That may have helped someone else, but it hadn't helped her enough.

Later, it emerged that part of what was keeping her stuck was this false image of me as so successful and accomplished. It was contributing to her fear of risking movement into some of the deeper vulnerabilities involved in her problems. How could she reveal her most despised parts of herself with such an elevated personage? Of course, it was also making her feel as if the impasse was all her fault. We were able to move on in our work together.

How did I grow? I learned, once again, that I don't have to know and do everything right. Instead, the main thing is to stay in the immediacy of the moment-to-moment movement of the relationship. Sometimes the way to do that is to put yourself at risk, to move into something new, even if in a small way. Of course, therapists should do so with thought and practice and should do something more considered than what I did here. The aim clearly is not to be careless or thoughtless.

We don't have to be able to predict and control everything. We can't do that anyhow. We do have to keep getting training and help from colleagues so that we are as knowledgeable and skillful as possible in what we do. Most important, we have to feel able to deal with "what happens next," to engage with whatever ensues, especially if we have made a major error or failure. This is where the most important work usually occurs. Sometimes, it is not as bad as our own CIs, RIs, and SDs have led us to fear. At best, we find that we are able to connect in new and enlarged ways.

Incidentally, this example may suggest projective identification. That is not the point I want to make. Pam was very conscious of feeling helpless. I would focus, instead, on the ways in which patient and therapist can find moment-to-moment movement toward better connection and also that this movement is mutual.

POWER

The third and more overriding point about change in therapy concerns the recognition of the importance of the patient's effect on the relationship and on the therapist. This notion is really implicit in the first point in the above list of recommendations for therapy–that is, that the therapist must feel with the patient and the patient must feel the therapist feeling with her. If this occurs, the patient must have had an effect on the therapist and on the relationship. However, we have not examined this effect thoroughly. More specifically, I'd like to explore the obstacles to movement-in-relationship that occur when the impact of the patient or the therapist turns to "power-over" forms of action rather than mutual empowerment.

We should note that the field of psychology has left the whole issue of power relatively underdeveloped. Alfred Adler raised it early but he was soon cast out by Freud and so was the whole topic.

Why is this issue so important? Actually, we and others are really saying that all psychological troubles arise because we haven't been able to affect the important relationships in our lives. We couldn't reach the other person(s) or couldn't bring about change in something that hurt. Even as infants, we affect our relationships as recent research has demonstrated. For example, Edward Tronick has produced striking videos that show infants trying to relate to their caretakers (1998). If the caretaker does not respond appropriately, the babies try several times more, but if a response does not occur, they turn away. These videos seem an amazing portrayal of exactly what we're talking about. The infant desires and seeks connection. When it seems impossible, s/he turns to disconnection, isolation. Of course, the strategies of disconnection become ever more complicated as the person goes on in life.

From earliest life, then, we should have an influence on the relationships in our lives just because of our thoughts and feelings. They should matter. Others should respond to them (which doesn't mean agree) and care about them. This is basic to the possibility of participating in relationships: if you are not having an effect on the relationship and the other people in it, you cannot really be participating in the relationship.

Thus, in therapy people have to regain a belief that they can have an influence on their relationships, beginning with the therapy relationship. Therapist and patient each affect the other and each must recognize and acknowledge this effect. Judy Jordan has written about this topic in her work on relational competence (1996). I am exploring the topic from the perspective of power.

There are additional immediate reasons why this matters in therapy. It is terrible to be in a room with someone and to feel one can't have an effect on her/him. How can you be safe? It's as if you are totally at the mercy of the other person. This point may relate to the point Amy Banks made that people suffering with chronic post traumatic stress disorder (PT SD) sometimes find it unbearable even to be in a room with a therapist (2000). She suggests that they are triggered to have the sort of brain chemical reactions that began when they were powerless when confronted by a perpetrator.

Traditionally, therapists have been encouraged to demonstrate that patients had no impact on them–that is, to not react to patients' thoughts and feelings. Therapists called on Freud's dictum that the analyst should display an "even hovering attention." At it's best, this advice admonished therapists to be nonjudgmental and not to "reward" or encourage one of the patient's utterances over another by showing more of a reaction to it. Some writers, even recently, have spoken of this attitude of giving patients this freedom and scope as a loving stance.

Instead, I believe this stance can lead to what is then labeled "acting out," as the patient attempts to elicit the therapist's response. Further, patient and therapist do inevitably affect each other. The point is to recognize this influence and to move in relationship toward affecting each other in ways that are mutually empathic and mutually empowering. Incidentally, Irene Stiver described an observation that she and many others who do many consultations know, that patients know accurately a great deal about their therapists' reactions. They have usually not told their therapists because they also pick up the notion that they should not be aware of what is going on (personal communication, 1991).

Patients are always trying to have an effect on their therapist. If they can't do so directly, their attempts will come in the form of strategies of disconnection. Some strategies may not look like attempts to have an effect, e.g., silences, intellectualizing, talking off the point, attack, anger, criticizing the therapist. There are many more. These strategies are also uses of power in that they prevent the relationship from moving, they create obstacles to movement. They certainly affect the therapist, but all of these actions are usually not conscious attempts to wield power.

On the therapist's part, she possesses more power than the patient as detailed below. Even so, there are times when the therapist feels threatened and not safe. Many of these instances follow from the controlling images we develop about ourselves as therapists, as Maureen Walker suggested (2001). This is what was happening to me in the example with Pam above. Therapists' CIs may include having to be all knowing and always competent. (Our RCT, if misunderstood, runs the risk of adding even more CIs such as we should be all empathic, all understanding, and the like.) These therapy CIs usually build on our particular cultural CIs and RIs such as believing we had to take care of everything, to solve all the family's problems, and others.

Threats to our CIs usually occur when therapy is not going well, often when we feel the patient is explicitly or implicitly making us feel pressured to make something improve or solve something. A good example of this kind of a moment occurs in the teaching video, entitled *Martha*, that Judy Jordan and a trainee role-played (Jordan & Lesses, 1998). They were trying to portray a disconnection. It began when the "patient" was pressing Judy to come up with a solution to her immobilization. Judy made a suggestion and the patient became very angry and sarcastic.

At these moments of disconnection I believe that we, as therapists, can ask ourselves the question: "Is it important to try to repair the relationship or is it important to try to repair some image of myself? Further, when we try to recoup some image of ourselves, we tend to fall back on some maneuver that is a power-over attempt. For example, in the video, Judy might have said, "I see you're angry. I am just trying to help." On the surface seemingly innocuous but indeed very disconnecting and a true put-down.

Why do we fall back on a power-over maneuver? Because that is what we learn in our culture. As Maureen Walker has captured it so well, "It is our default position." Because that is how our society is structured and how we all tend to respond. It can happen in a split second and usually without our awareness. Thus, the whole power-over mode of acting enters the therapy room. In this sense, we can see therapy as a realm in which we are trying to learn a new way of relating, different from that of our dominant culture.

In the example with my patient Pam, she saved me from the attempt to try to repair my images by making it easy for me to say that I often felt helpless and, most important, she also made it possible for me to affirm my belief in this process. The latter helped me counter the discouragement I had introduced.

Judy's response in the video illustrates a much better way of moving into connection. Judy says that she felt the patient didn't like what she (Judy) said, and it made her (the patient) angry. "And I felt bad," says Judy. This response led them back into very good movement. Note that this is not therapist's authenticity for the sake of "disclosure." It is an authentic statement that moves the relationship into connection. Further, Judy tells the patient that she cares about her and about the relationship. The patient has an effect on Judy and it matters to her.

This video also portrays a growing point for the therapist as well as the patient, that is, it illustrates mutuality. Such moments lead us to stretch, to do something new, not because the patient is there to help us grow but because we have tried to move the relationship toward better connection, toward the goal of therapy. When we participate in that process, we also grow. None of us get it right all of the time and on the spot. We do get second chances, and sometimes third and fourth.

Even to ask the question, "What am I trying to repair here?" may help us to move to a new track. It can create a pause in our automatic response to repair our own images. We will return to this point in the next section.

After working on this talk for a while, I realized that this section is really spelling out in a little more detail some of the specific components in impasses that Irene Stiver wrote about in her paper, *A Relational Approach to Therapeutic Impasses* (1990). In that brilliant paper, she said that impasses occur when the patient feels disconnected from the therapist and the therapist follows by disconnecting from the patient. The therapist is usually not aware of what's happening initially. It makes me happy to be carrying forward her work in this way.

WHAT TO DO?

What to do? The answer lies in working toward increasing the patient's affect on the relationship and toward the patient's and the therapist's recognition and acknowledgment of that effect. As a first step, we can recognize how the whole therapy arrangement augments the therapist's power. We and others have written about this (Miller & Stiver, 1997); so I will just review some of the features. The patient is the person coming with problems; she is in the supplicant position. To be in this position immediately makes her feel "one-down" in our culture. While this should not be true, it is how people are made to feel. We don't have good models of a helping relationship that is respectful and empowering for the help seeker. Our difficulty in finding a word for the seeker reflects this situation. We have struggled over not liking either the words, patient or client for years and have not found a good word in our common language.

The patient comes to the therapist; she is stepping into the therapist's domain as Wendy Rosen said (2002). Once there, the therapist sets the whole frame, it is usually quite rigid and not to be questioned. The patient is supposed to be more exposed psychologically, more vulnerable. She is always in the "helped" position, never the helper or equal contributor; this situation usually makes a person feel inferior and less empowered. Very often the way we present ourselves leads patients to feel less powerful. For example, we appear as professionals, often of high status, all knowing with all of our problems solved as Judy Jordan says (1998).

Most important the patient usually feels she cares more than the therapist. In truth, we may matter more to patients than they do to us. However, as discussed earlier, patients and our relationships with them also do matter to us although traditionally, we have not let them know this. This situation may create the most important power differential of all. The person who cares the most usually feels at a great disadvantage in power. Further, this feeling usually leads to serious shame, which then increases a person's sense of powerlessness, silence, and difficulty representing her experience.

As in transference, patients can see the therapist as similar to those powerful people in the past whom she would not be able to affect, to reach. But the therapist has more power and status, in fact, in the present. This power differential will become more complex if the patient is from a group defined as "lesser than" by the society.

Thus, the therapy situation, itself, tends to increase a patient's strategies of disconnection because of this power difference. Traditionally, therapists have talked of therapy creating dependency but have not considered extensively the creation of powerlessness.

Further, structural factors in reality may operate to give the therapist significant real power over the patients' lives, for example, in institutionalized patients and in some managed care arrangements. Elizabeth Sparks made this point about her work with adolescents remained to an institution by the court. Her suggestion is to acknowledge the truth and to honor the fact that she is struggling with these reality constraints (2001). Denying and mystifying power is the worst course and one that we know is common to those in power-over positions.

INITIAL SESSION

Having recognized this major power differential, what steps can we take? We can very consciously work to make this differential clear and to increase the patient's power. This action can start with the very first interview with steps like the following: We can explain how we work and ask what the patient expects. Sometimes people expect something very different and it is best to discuss that. Second, we can explain the conditions in which we can work. We can say, "You tell me what you'd like" and try to meet the patient's conditions. When we can't, we should be honest about it.

As part of the way we work, we can explain that this work depends on a dialogue, an interaction based on mutuality, with words like, "I can't possibly do it alone." This kind of mutual engagement may be different from what the patient is accustomed to in other healing situations. Cultural characteristics may enter here and the therapist may have to deal more extensively with the differences from the patient's expectations.

It is important to urge patients to ask questions and to say that asking them truly will help the work. They keep the therapist more in touch with the patient's experience. We can say that we will answer questions when we feel able but may not do so if it makes us too uncomfortable. We can also ask the patient to tell us as the work goes along when we are not getting the point or not being responsive.

I'm sure we can think of additional suggestions. Although specifics are important, the most significant feature is that they convey an attitude of openness, of the therapist's desire to hear the patient, and wish to change when the relationship calls for it. They can create a tone that will help to increase the patient's influence on the work. This mode is very different from the old model of the expert "acting on" the patient.

AS THERAPY PROCEEDS

As therapy proceeds, perhaps we should consider the possibility that another central guide may be that we act always to increase the patient's influence on the relationship and accordingly, to increase the patient's awareness of her influence. We might consider this focus another key goal that we should pursue throughout. Although considering it at all times, it may be especially important at the moments when we are feeling disconnected. Can it be that we, as therapists, have resisted the patient's influence and she's felt she had to turn to her strategies of disconnection. Or have we, as therapists, done something that is making the patient feel our excess power, perhaps without awareness.

To try to attend to this possibility, we can, again, first of all, try to be open to it. This openness may be most important when working with people of marginalized groups but it is important with everyone. Just being aware of these possibilities can change us. It changes what we're inclined to say next as opposed to blithely going on our way as if this possibility didn't exist.

Further, when we feel something is occurring that we may not understand, we can ask about it. For example, one patient was going through a very difficult period at her job. She was overworked, stressed and complaining about it. I felt her workplace was very unfair and I said something like, "That's so hard. You must be very tired." Empathic? No. (Note that the last comment is not a good thing to say ever. It is not wise to tell people what they must be feeling.) The exchange stopped for a fleeting moment. I said, "Did I say something you didn't like." She said, "Oh no, of course not." However, this brief exchange did open up a possibility that she became able to talk about later. It turned out that in her family she had to accomplish everything perfectly and do so while always looking healthy and beautiful. To accomplish this feat gave her some power and influence with parents whom she often felt were out of reach. My comment made her feel drained of her accustomed source of effectiveness in relationships but asking her about her reaction felt like a first step in opening up a very charged topic. At the time she didn't have clarity about it and neither did I. However, she later said that my asking created the first slight glimmer of light in a very obscure and confusing area. For the first time, she felt a small belief that this whole topic could even be talked about.

Another way patients can recognize their effect on the relationship occurs when we tell our responses. This kind of comment depends a great deal on the stage of the relationship and must be done with wise attention to what will help to move the relationship forward. The example from the video above is a very good one (Jordan & Lesses, 1998).

We can't always talk about the relationship directly because that is often one of the most difficult things for patients to do–and for therapists as well. Again, it can help just to be aware or questioning of our own feelings. We can also address this issue in ways that don't entail talking about the relationship directly, e.g., by asking a question such as, "Is there something I'm not getting now?" Thus, it's not always a question of telling our reactions as they arise but of using them to try to question whether a power-over dynamic is at play, one that the patient may not be able to get at. Jan Surrey made the point in discussing the *Martha* video that the patient may feel less powerful based on the status factors at play (2001). Martha sees Judy as a professional in a high status job compared to herself, who can't even get a job. Further, she sees Judy as thin, therefore much "better than" she according to the controlling images in this society. Jan makes the point that often a patient's anger and criticism can be based on such sources of power difference. Indeed, they can be understood as attempts at authenticity although the patient cannot state them directly. They may be a way of saying, "Something is wrong in this relationship." Jan adds that she learned this in working with patients and therapists of marginalized groups.

EXPERTISE

Since I have emphasized the importance of the patient's influence on the therapeutic relationship, a question may arise about the place of the therapist's expertise. Aren't therapists supposed to know and do something more than the patient does? Therapists absolutely need great expertise but it's a question of the *kind* of expertise–and the kind of expertise that offers the most safeguard against power-over actions. That expertise consists of the ability to participate in movement-in-relationship toward better connection, as stated at the beginning. This kind of expertise requires profound abilities; it is complex and can be very difficult. It requires extensive training and continuing help from colleagues. Further, the therapist has to have a grounding in knowledge of psychological functioning and development.

While the therapist requires this kind of expertise, the patient possesses certain kinds of knowledge that the therapist can never have. Only the patient knows what happened in her experience and how it led her to construct controlling images, relational images and strategies of disconnection–and especially, the clues to how she can move into better connection. She does not know all of this consciously but only she can supply both the steps and the obstacles to bringing them into the relationship and to changing them. She can gain access to them only as you work together.

In her study applying RCT to the workplace, Joyce Fletcher coined the term "fluid expertise" (1999). She meant that knowledge and ability can flow back and forth between and among workers; and between workers and supervisors. As one of the women she interviewed said, "No one knows it all." Encouraging fluid expertise can lead to all workers becoming more empowered and creative.

The term applies to therapy and yet we're dealing with a more complex interchange. There are powerful forces keeping patients from knowing what only they know. Thus, the true expertise lies in increasing our ability to find the paths to both patient and therapist participating in the relationship so that it moves toward better connection. This increased connection leads to the patient bringing into the relationship more and more of her experience and becoming more able to examine her CIs, RIs and SDs. This, in turn, leads to more connection, which leads to bringing more experience into the relationship and so on in a spiraling interchange of growth.

CONCLUSION

As therapists, most of us, I believe, want a world where everyone can change and grow. For that, we need to change whatever societal forces keep anyone from growing. This is a tall order. Another concept of Patricia Hill Collins (2000) has helped me think about this tall order. She writes of the term, "visionary pragmatist." She uses it to describe how African American women contributed to African American society beginning before the Civil Rights Movement. They played a major part in the growth and protection of their children, but not only their own children those of family, neighbors, friends, and in the neighborhood in general. They participated in the church and in other organizations and institutions. By the very way they lived, these women enacted a vision that went beyond the current situation.

These women contributed to the growth of people and institutions in day-to-day life even as they were aware of the power structure that affected them and even if they could not change the whole system. They were pragmatists. But they were living by a morality and a value system that was different and more advanced. They were living by a different vision. Many were ready to make greater change when that possibility came about, for example, Fanny Lou Hamer, Rosa Parks, and many others whose names most people don't even know.

I don't mean to suggest that privileged middle-class therapists of today are the same at all. But I do think we can learn from that concept; know the importance of holding a vision and finding ways to practice it even in current life, while building toward larger change. Indeed, I believe that if we are truly helping people to change and grow, we are inevitably moving in a way that counters the restrictive CIs of society.

Patricia Hill Collins' concepts may provide an additional example of how mutuality proceeds in a system. She evolved these ideas out of the truth of her experience as a woman of a marginalized group in this society. When people of marginalized groups tell the truth of their experience, they open up and illuminate the truth about the dominant group as well–and about the whole system. For example, we can see how controlling images affect everyone. They are not the same controlling image for all social groups but they help us see and understand the total society in a fuller and truer light. And this larger view can contribute to us all and to helping us make change in the system.

Despite dwelling on the problems of change, which we must continue to do as therapists–and as people who have a vision of a better world, I want to reiterate that I believe change–growth–is the most essential and exhilarating thing about living. All people are seeking it. It is our task to keep finding better ways to participate in this process.

REFERENCES

Banks, A. (2000, April). *The Neurobiology of Traumatic Disconnection.* Paper presented at the Learning from Women Conference, co-sponsored by Harvard Medical School/Cambridge Hospital and the Jean Baker Miller Training Institute, Boston, MA.

Collins, P. H. (2000). *Black feminist thought* (2nd ed.). New York: Routledge.

Fletcher, J. K. (1999). *Disappearing acts: Gender, power, and relational practice at work.* Cambridge, MA: MIT Press.

Jordan, J. (1996). Toward connection and competence. *Work in Progress, No. 83.* Wellesley, MA: Stone Center Working Paper Series.

Jordan, J. (1998). Clinical Vignettes: "Martha." *Videotape, No. 5.* Wellesley, MA: Stone Center Working Paper Series.

Jordan, J. (1998). Personal Communication.

Miller, J. B. (1988). Connections, disconnections, and violations. *Work in Progress, No. 33.* Wellesley, MA: Stone Center Working Paper Series.

Miller, J. B., & Stiver, I. P. (1997). *The healing connection.* Boston: Beacon Press.

Rapoport, R., Bailyn, L., Fletcher, J. K., & Pruitt, B. H. (2002). *Beyond work-family balance: Advancing gender equity and workplace performance.* San Francisco: Jossey-Bass.

Sparks, E. (1998). Against all odds: Resistance and resilience in African American welfare mothers. *Work in Progress, No. 81.* Wellesley, MA: Stone Center Working Paper Series.

Sparks, E. (2001). Personal Communication.

Stiver, I. (1990). A relational approach to therapeutic impasses. *Work in Progress No. 58.* Wellesley, MA: Stone Center Working Paper Series.

Stiver, I. P., Rosen, W. B., Surrey, J., & Miller, J. B. (2000). Creative moments in relational-cultural therapy. *Work in Progress, No. 92.* Wellesley, MA: Stone Center Working Paper Series.

Surrey, J. (2001, October). Founding Concepts/Recent Developments in Relational-Cultural Theory [comments during large group discussion]. Jean Baker Miller Fall Intensive Training Institute, Dover, MA.

Tronick, E. (1998). Dyadically expanded states of consciousness and the process of therapeutic change. *Infant Mental Health Journal, 19*(3), 290-299.

Walker, M. (2001). Presentation at Jean Baker Miller Summer Intensive Training Institute, Wellesley, MA.

Walker, M., & Miller, J. B. (2000). Racial images and relational possibilities. *Talking Paper, No. 2.* Wellelsey, MA: Stone Center Working Paper Series.

Power and Effectiveness: Envisioning an Alternate Paradigm

Maureen Walker

SUMMARY. Relational-Cultural Theory provides a straightforward and elegant definition of power; it is the capacity to produce change. The implication of this framework is that power is the energy of competence in everyday living. However, in a culture stratified along multiple dimensions–race, class, and sexual orientation to name a few–power is associated with hyper-competitiveness and deterministic control. The article begins by examining the "protective illusions" of the power-over paradigm, where humanity is rank ordered according to perceived cultural value and is stratified into groups of greater than and less than. In addition to exposing the false dichotomies of power-over arrangements, the article examines the destructive consequences of cultural disconnection, on both the putative winners and the losers. Examples from organizational practice, clinical relationships, and socio-political contexts are used to illustrate the Relational-Cultural Model in action. Specifically, scenarios are presented from the standpoint of the politically disempowered to demonstrate the relational competencies of empathic attunement,

---

Maureen Walker, PhD, is Director of Program Development, JBMTI; Associate Director of Support Services, Harvard Business School; in private practice for psychotherapy and multicultural consultation, Cambridge, MA; and co-editor of *How Connections Heal* and *The Complexity of Connection*.

authenticity, and accountability that foster healing, resilience, and mutual empowerment. This article was originally presented at the 2002 Spring Training Institute sponsored by the Jean Baker Miller Training Institute at Wellesley College.

INTRODUCTION

There is probably a no more straightforward and elegant definition of power than that proposed by Jean Baker Miller: Power is the capacity to produce change (1991). This definition suggests that power is a fundamental energy of everyday living. However, in a culture that valorizes radical individualism (Jordan, 2002), power is associated with hyper-competitiveness, conquest, and might. Power mutates into "power-over," and is then viewed as the entitlement of the "winners"–those individuals who have attained the social ranking and the material accoutrements that signify value. Such a model is quite impoverished. Envisioning a more inclusive model begins with acts of revelation: bringing to light the stories and experiences of those people who are typically characterized as vulnerable and marginalized, people who are seen as the "losers" in a power-over paradigm. What these stories often reveal are everyday strategies of attunement, empathy, and reciprocity that not only enable survival, but also enlarge capacity for navigating the complex illusions and machinations of power-over social arrangements.

One such story involves my memory of a power negotiation that occurred on an ordinary Saturday morning well over 40 years ago. On this particular Saturday morning, my mother and I walked into downtown Augusta, Georgia to pay the rent on 1131 Summer Street, the three-room clapboard structure that was my home for at least the first ten years of my life. When we entered the Lucky Real Estate office, my mother presented her cash payment (cash she had earned providing domestic service for white families) to the white woman behind the counter.

When my mother counted her cash and put it on the counter, this woman who did not know my mother, pushed it back at her and said, "Mary, you need to go and get some change." The racial context of this encounter is significant for two reasons. First, only white people–usually women–worked behind counters in downtown offices in Augusta in the

1950s. Second, although she did not know my mother, any white woman could, and was in fact *expected* to, exercise the entitlement of familiarity, calling my mother by her first name only to signify the difference in their social ranking. Knowing my mother as I do now, I doubt that she even blinked. I do remember her asking very calmly: "*Who needs to go and get some change?*" I think there were several moments of silence because no one spoke another word. The woman picked up the money, gave my mother proper change and our rent receipt. We then left and went about the business of doing whatever the two of us did on Saturday mornings.

It seems to me that those of us who occupy positions of relative privilege have much to learn from those who occupy the bottom strata of the dominant power hierarchy. In fact, the historical failure of mainstream feminist movements has been the manifest and compound exclusion of women subjugated by race and class in the dominant power arrangements. It is from these people that we can draw insight and inspiration for visions of alternative paradigms. Alice Walker's fictional character Janie Crawford is an example of such a woman (1979).

It occurs to me that a part of my attraction to Janie Crawford (and women like her) is that she subverts the restrictive fictions of a power-over paradigm, choosing how she will relate to a social structure that would limit her life to dichotomous choices.

From the founding concepts to the more recent formulations, Relational-Cultural Theory has grappled with issues of power. I consciously use the word grapple because it connotes collective struggle, political risk, and interpersonal discomfort. Jean Baker Miller (1987) laid the foundation for this struggle in her book, *Toward a New Psychology of Women*, when she stated that:

> In most instances of difference, there is also a factor of inequality–inequality of many kinds of resources, but fundamentally of status and power. These inequalities, which are often natural and essential, all too often mutate into power-over relationships . . . relationships in which there is no assumption that the goal of the relationship is to end the inequality.

Miller elaborates on this point by commenting that in fact, quite the reverse happens. The dominant group is the model for "normal" relationships. It then becomes "normal" to treat those with less power destructively to obscure the truth of that destructiveness, and to oppose any movement toward equality. In most contemporary social structures, including but not limited to modern work places, rigid stratification of power not only looks normal, it begins to feel necessary. Thus the everyday mystifications that support distorted power arrangements achieve operational credibility, and through practices of either cultural extortion or seduction, they cloud our vision and enervate our capacity for productive critique. In other words, through either the threat of exclusion and/or annihilation, or the illusory promise of inclusion and/or protection, the dominant power arrangements co-opt the talents of the most well-intentioned among us in order to maintain and reproduce their own interests. They do so by quieting the voices of opposition–the voices that would question the foundational values upon which hierarchical power rests.

Elizabeth Janeway (1980) describes our cultural legacy of power similarly:

> Power, as we have seen it, involves mastery, with its connotations of individual might, heroic stature, lone suffering that must win, perhaps, a solution born of the mind of a single genius who has achieved a new vision.

Using a term coined by Bernard Loomer, Rita Nakashima Brock (1993) writes that "unilateral power" presupposes an ego-centered, self-contained person, one who aims at creating the largest determining effect on others, while being minimally influenced by the other. Not coincidentally, this model of power is totally congruent with the model that traditional psychology sets forth as "the healthy self," a self of firmly bounded independence guided by its internal locus of control (Jordan, 1991). This paradigm of power, like this paradigm of self, is grounded in either-or choices. This paradigm of power–like this paradigm of self–is based upon what Karen Brodkin (1998) calls the "social binary," where "difference" devolves into better than or worse than and "different from" is translated as "opposition to." In this system, power is a commodity to be owned, increased, and used over and against those who threaten its reproduction. People who accrue more of this commodity are deemed more valuable. In such a paradigm, power functions to cement into place inequality between dominants and subordinates.

Given that legacy, it is small wonder that people who have been historically marginalized (e.g., women) are often observed to be uncomfortable with power. Contrary to traditional wisdom, this discomfort has less to do with women's inadequacies and more to do with the flaws of the dominant paradigm.

Miller (1991) has noted that dominating power, or what we call "the power-over factor" results in women equating power with selfishness, destructiveness, and ultimately abandonment. However, I would also submit that in part, ambivalence about power can lead to reproducing its most destructive arrangements and consequences.

It was my fascination with notions of power and fear of success that led to my doctoral dissertation research. I was fascinated largely because I was drawn to the work of Karen Horney and because I witnessed the ravages of ambivalence and relational distortion in the lives of very successful women all around me. I was interested to know what happened in women's intimate relationships when they are publicly perceived as powerful. Once in a chance conversation with a faculty member I mentioned the name of an African American woman on my committee. He commented with undisguised derision that this woman probably made an excellent committee member. "After all," he said, "she managed to get tenure, but she still goes home alone every night and eats cold cereal." More recently, young professional women commented on a national news magazine show that they took great care to hide the fact that they attended a prestigious graduate school of management if they hoped to meet potential dating partners. The power-over culture renders false dichotomies, reducing and constricting the range of human potential. This paradigm offers the possibility to dominate or be dominated; to be successful or to be alone; to be mule or queen.

To envision an alternative paradigm is to reject the false dichotomies of the dominant paradigm in favor of a more complex, fully inhabited experience of relationship.

Consistent with Miller's assertion that power is the capacity to facilitate movement, Brock (1993) wrote in *Journeys by Heart* that persons in our society feel present, alive, and sustained in the world through power–power to influence and participate in shaping the world. Power, she maintains, is a basic human reality precisely *because* we are related to each other. If the goal of relationship is movement and creativity, then embracing power is a necessary function. To disavow power is not an option. The option is to choose how to relate *to* and *through* the power that one has.

To disavow power is to disavow relational accountability. In fact, disavowal and denial are preferred tactics for protecting the status quo in power-over arrangements. By suppressing the conflict that could potentially transform the infrastructure of power, and by obscuring the reality of its tactics, these arrangements continually reproduce their own interests. An example from the workplace illustrates the point. A new manager was assigned to a department in which the relationships at their best could be described as contentious. She began her first meeting by announcing the new departmental norms: trust, mutual respect, and open communication. As this example suggests, good intentions don't automatically translate into good use of power. The goals and intentions may in fact be noble or benign. However, when motives toward deterministic control lie at the base of those intentions, movement toward clarity and mutuality in relationship will be compromised.

Brock (1993) maintains that it is for this reason that we should turn to the vulnerable to study power, that is, to turn to those who have least access to cultural commodities or affirmation to study power. Limiting our attention to those who are perceived as strong, the benefactors and the beneficiaries of the dominant paradigm, can lead to a distorted view of power. I am reminded of a group exercise called "The Privilege Walk" that those of us who have traveled the diversity circuit have probably encountered. In this exercise, participants get to take steps forward or backward depending upon their relationship to a number of socially constructed factors: gender, physical ability, location in the economic structures, etc. Steps forward represent participation in arenas of privilege, while steps backward represent areas of disadvantage. Obviously as the game progresses, those participants with compounded privilege (e.g., white, male, upper-class, heterosexual, physically able, etc.) are so far ahead that they can literally only see what's in front of them. The Saturday morning encounter in the Lucky Real Estate office also richly illustrates this point. My mother worked as a domestic for $20 a week. At that time, she had neither property, nor education, nor marriage to a man–none of the cultural accoutrements that would validate her worth as a human being. She only had that moment in relationship–a moment in which she chose to fully inhabit her aliveness and her dignity.

My mother's and my economic survival and physical safety depended upon her attunement to the relational co-surround in relationship to my mother; the woman behind the desk was the face of power. My mother had to be aware of her standing in relationship to the woman, where the woman stood vis-à-vis her own boss, and consequences of aggravated conflict with the woman. In this particular power context, the choices would *appear* to be limited: to succumb to humiliation at the hands of another woman who was trying to put her in her place or to compound her victimization by indulging fantasies of domination. Either choice would have been a strategy of profound disconnection. To paraphrase an idea put forth by bell hooks (2000) in *Margin to Center*, to adopt the values of the dominant power paradigm is to impoverish our choices. Karen Kollias (1975) goes on to explain:

While middle-class models of power, have primarily been white men, lower-and working-class women, especially non-white women, have seldom been able to depend on someone else for their decisions and maintenance. The process of taking active control over their lives and influencing those close to them has given them a lifetime of experience with decision-making of the most basic nature: survival.

To make visible the experiences of marginalized women in exploring the complex potentialities of power is to enact the feminist principles of relationship and a reversal in our scholarship: to create theory "from the ground up."

Miller (1987) echoed these principles when she asserted that dominant, deterministic power obscures the realities of relationship. It affects the appearance of lone, individualistic action when, in fact, action is supported by an entire system. Fletcher, Jordan, and Miller (2000) explained that these supports are interwoven in the very fabric of being and are thereby invisible. All power, including destructive power, is created by and depends upon relationship. When we believe the lie of lone individualism, women–and all people who do not have access to the invisible supports–are left feeling deficient, or are somehow labeled less competent or less committed in systems where power distortions are the norm.

A few decades ago, the self-help industry set out to rectify this deficiency by producing a spate of publications all designed to help women become better, more enthusiastic mimics of the mythical, self-contained (self-made) man and exercise some version of mythical self-contained power. The shelves were filled with such titles: everything from *Games Your Mother Never Taught You* and *The Cinderella Complex* to *Dress for Success*. Recently, I have seen at least two popular magazines urging women to mimic men in order to wrest power and control in their work lives. This advice about hoarding power was dispensed not only to women engaged in business enterprises but also to those of us in mental health professions. In one videotaped session after another, students are admonished not to engage in power struggles with their clients, with simultaneous warnings about the dire consequences that would ensue should we ever leak our power out of the therapeutic frame to the client. In other words, we were taught to win by pretending that we were not engaged in battle. We were taught to engage power by obscuring reality and lying–I think even or perhaps especially–to ourselves. The paradigm of hierarchical, ego-bounded power is grounded in reactive fearfulness of zero-sum choices, in which we must gain power-over to avoid being overpowered. Such power cannot be embraced; it can only be temporarily extorted.

ENVISIONING AN ALTERNATIVE PARADIGM

Two questions that support the process of envisioning an alternative paradigm of power are the following:

1. If power is a fundamental energy of relationship, how does power look when used in service of zest, clarity, mutuality, and affirmation of connection?
2. How might our relationship with power help us to more fully inhabit our lives?

Brock (1993) suggests that we begin by thinking of power as ambiguous and open-ended. She speaks of power as processes that create and sustain relationship; she also describes power as bonds that are created and sustained by our relational selves.

RELATIONAL CONFLICT

A telling indicator of how we embrace power is how we engage conflict. Which leads to another founding principle of Relational-Cultural Theory: that conflict is necessary for growth (Miller, 1987). Under the power-over paradigm, the dominant group moves expeditiously to suppress conflict precisely because its interests are served when the status quo can be represented as consensus. The oppressed group might likewise participate in this arrangement through a variety of disconnection strategies: from mimicking the postures and practices of the dominant group or by disavowing their own power and relevance in relationship. Again, these are strategies of disconnection that result from accepting the reductionist terms of the power-over paradigm. To embrace power from a relational perspective is to enlarge the terms of engagement. Most often, it means creating a new choice out of the dichotomized options.

COMBINING "OPPOSITES"

Let me share a case in point. In one of her early talks, Irene Stiver (1991) recounted an incident in which she tried to discuss an issue that for her was quite emotionally charged with a male colleague. As the conversation wore on, the intensity of her feelings grew. The more intense her feelings, the more agitated, unavailable, and dismissive he became. She eventually decided to take a different tack. She stripped the emotional color from the content and coolly recited the facts, to which he exclaimed, "Well why didn't you say so?" He went on to chide her for "coming on like a witch on a broom." Stiver pointed out that her emotion was a very important part of her content; yet, the incident is an all too familiar rendering of the dichotomous choices offered up by patriarchal power paradigms. One is either rational or emotional, professional or (the word that most expeditiously silences most women) unprofessional. This incident poignantly illustrates Jordan's (1991) assertion that underlying the prevailing models of power is the belief that affect is incompatible with cognitive effectiveness. Further, cognition is not only different from affect; it is superior and in opposition to affect. For that reason, women come to believe that emotions are to be hidden, disposed of, or at the very least neutralized.

A recent conversation with a client (let's call her Ellie) serves to illustrate this point. Ellie is Ivy League educated with a degree in business; she is also a woman with psychiatric disabilities. She has spent the last six years of her life working in various clerical "temp" assignments. In describing an encounter with her supervisor over a missed deadline, she commented that she felt inept at explaining a technical process to her impatient supervisor. Ellie was very aware that positionally she was the least powerful, most expendable member of the team. When I asked her how she felt when the supervisor approached her with an impatient, accusatory tone, she at first said she didn't know. Eventually she was able to name her feelings of guilt, annoyance, and embarrassment. She then resumed talking about how inadequate she felt trying to explain herself. I then asked her how she felt about that at the time. She immediately said, "I don't think I felt anything, but I believe I knew I had a right to them." I then asked: "If you can imagine your feelings as a physical object, what would it be?" Eventually she said her feelings were rather like a wall. I asked if we could imagine her feelings as a door, an opening through which to reach another person. She immediately responded that she would never want the supervisor to know that she felt guilty. "So your guilty feelings–and the others–could potentially endanger you in some way?" "Absolutely." The conversation went on: "It's pretty hard to feel friendly toward some aspect of yourself that could imperil you?" "Right . . . I try to hide them right away." In her desperation, the only solution she could imagine was to disconnect from her feeling-thoughts–and after years of socialization, this happened almost automatically.

As we talked, it was clear that this woman felt trapped in a dichotomy. The big question, the *only* question this dichotomy allowed her, was should she or should she not *express* her feelings in a professional setting. Following from that dichotomy is a series of corollary falsehoods. For example, that there is only one way to experience and express frustration, guilt, sadness, or excitement; that frustration causes outburst; that sadness equals weeping; that excitement creates frenzy.

We decided that one way to enlarge her operational space was to include more options; the question then became how I will relate to all of the feelings I'm having. She was able to stay connected to her feeling-thoughts and begin to generate options out of them. She decided that there was something essentially true, meaningful, and useful in each of her feelings, and that it was actually the *conflict,* her encounter with her supervisor, that raised those realities to light. Her supervisor, first an antagonist, became a potential ally. She then came up with an action plan for future encounters: first, to breathe and if not welcome her feelings to at least treat them politely as one might an unexpected guest; to acknowledge the supervisor's concerns; to address the problem in whatever way seems appropriate; and to invite suggestions. In many ways, Ellie was learning to embrace power by combining opposites. She recognized that the restrictive categories of the dominant paradigm that kept her from fully inhabiting her experience also restricted her range of motion and action in relationship. She decided to engage conflict by trying on the role of what Harriet Rubin (1998) calls the "collaborative antagonist." From a place of connection with her own feeling-thoughts, Ellie felt empowered to risk empathic attunement with her supervisor. And from that place of mutual empathy, she was more open to the kind of learning that facilitated both her own growth and the accomplishment of organizational goals.

Learning to engage collaborative conflict is critical to the relational exercise of power. Moreover, the context of collaborative conflict holds rich potential for exercise of power as energy, strength, and effective interaction.

CHOOSING RELATIONAL ACCOUNTABILITY

I have often spoken of a conflictual situation that occurred in my work life a few years ago. In brief, I was a part of a reorganization effort in which several new members were brought into the department. While I was the senior member of the team, I was not its leader and was feeling quite frustrated. I was being thwarted in my efforts to make the kinds of contributions that I was capable of and, in my view, *obliged* to make.

Once when someone asked me how I felt about my new team, I responded that *I felt like a lobster in a boiling pot*. The symbol speaks volumes–primarily about the relational images I carried into conflict and the strategies of disconnection I employed that served to exacerbate the distortions and hostilities thus foreclosing opportunities for movement. As relational images function to explain self, other, the purposes and the possibilities for relationship, a lobster that's already in a boiling pot has a fairly certain outcome. In spite of all of the clamoring and clanging about, at some point it's certain it's going to be somebody's dinner.

These images may then function to support a stance of victimness that justifies lack of relational accountability. Having declared myself the victim in this situation, I felt justified in some of my more clangorous "assertions." Had I fully internalized the lessons from my mother, I might have chosen differently–for to behave clangorously in most organizations is almost to ensure that you will become someone's dinner.

CHOOSING MUTUAL EMPOWERMENT

To engage in collaborative conflict is to relinquish any claim on the illusion of victory or power over another being. When the focus remains on mutual empowerment, there is little room for the instant gratification of tit-for-tat interactions. In other words, engaging in relational conflict requires relearning how to breathe, to reflect, and to connect with feeling-thoughts *before* attempting to influence the other person. It also means–and this is crucial–allowing oneself to be moved or influenced by another. (Recall the masterful, autonomous and bounded self resists external influence.)

Clearly under conditions of inequitable power and domination, the notion of mutual impact can feel quite threatening. In no way do I wish to minimize the oppression that many people in the world endure by blithely suggesting that they open themselves to being influenced by their oppressors. I am suggesting that those of us who do not live with the daily threat of subjugation and annihilation have more choices than the limited power-over paradigms would have us believe.

I think again of my mother's quiet but forceful query, which sought not to obliterate the woman behind the desk, but to subvert the power paradigm that defined my mother as an inferior being. Moreover, my mother refused to indulge those strategies of disconnection that ultimately result in self-obliteration. I am convinced that my mother made use of what Elizabeth Janeway (1980) calls the power of disbelief. She refused to believe the humiliating lies of the power-over paradigm; lies that defined her as less than human, unworthy of respect, or as Walker's (1919) character put it, "one of the mules of the world." I am also convinced that she gave the woman an opportunity to relinquish her image of the proper relationship between a white and a black woman, and the opportunity to pay more attention to the actual relationship she was living in the moment.

AMPLIFYING DIFFERENCE TO EXPAND THE RELATIONAL SPACE

The radical notion in the practice of relational power is that rather than constricting the antagonist to the role of adversary, it possible to engage conflict by embracing the difference, by engaging the point of view that the antagonist represents (Rubin, 1998). In *Margin to Center*, bell hooks speaks eloquently to this notion when she comments that women need the experience of working through conflict. Our socialization into the power-over paradigm would have us believe that in conflict our options are limited to victimizing or destroying. Often, because of our fear of intractable disconnection, we sabotage our chances for sustainable solidarity by offering instead the illusion of support.

The power-over paradigm would have us rush to common ground before fully engaging the rich potentialities of our differences. Interestingly, some of the more recent research on negotiation practices suggests that the rush to common ground results in an impoverished negotiation. To quote one management pundit, "rushing to common ground leaves way too much money on the table." The somewhat counter-intuitive notion is that amplifying differences can serve to enrich the relationship and unleash collaborative powers that might otherwise have remained constrained. From either side of the inequality there is the notion that any challenge to the *status quo* can only be dangerous.

The practice of relational conflict requires renunciation of the usual terms of power in that the antagonist is valued for her difference (however awkwardly it might be packaged), is listened into fuller voice, and encouraged to engage in deeper connection.

PRACTICING SUPPORTED VULNERABILITY

Relational conflict allows and is supported by the practice of courage in vulnerability. (I'm intrigued by the notion that within some contexts, we might practice softening ourselves for conflict instead of bracing ourselves for conflict . . . staying in the relationship connected to our own voice and as Jordan (2002) suggests "listening the other into voice.") A central tenet of Relational-Cultural Theory is that humans learn and grow through action in relationship by staying present, alive, and connected in the present moment, a place of profound vulnerability. I recently listened to a talk in which the speaker suggested that most organizations expect the employees to function like stealth fighters: steeled-strength, silent, functional, and, above all, invulnerable. The irony, according to Thomas (2002), is that it is in our vulnerability that we find our growing edge.

PRACTICING THE POWER OF NAMING

In addition to relational conflict, one of the practices that subverts the restrictive fictions of the power-over paradigm is the practice of complaint. The dominant powers attempt to suppress complaint, by any means necessary, but most often through humiliation and shaming (after all, we are told nobody likes a whiner). To complain, to publicly admit injury or weakness or harm is to disrupt the status quo. Miller (1987) calls this naming of injury "an act of vast exposure."

No one more dramatically embodies this principle than a woman named Mamie Bradley. Mrs. Bradley was a black mother whose son Emmet Till was murdered while vacationing in Mississippi because he allegedly whistled at a 27-year-old white woman. As the reports go, the woman's boyfriend and his friends shot 15-year-old Emmet in the head, tied a 70-pound block around his neck, and threw him into the Tallahatchie River. When his body was returned to his mother, she opened the coffin and wept publicly on the platform of a Chicago train station. Instead of hiding the ugliness, pain, and horror of what happened, she chose another course. She allowed journalists to take photographs of his mutilated body. She delayed the funeral for days so that thousands of people could visit the funeral home and "see what had been done to her boy."

Hers was a powerful act of resistance in a culture that would shame her into hiding and silence. Many were moved to action as a result of seeing the photographs of the mutilated corpse and hearing his mother talk. Mamie Bradley decided to go back to school. In her own words: "my burning thing, the thing that has come out of Emmet's death is to learn until your head swells." She made a clear distinction between resistance and hatred. She went on, "I did not spend one minute hating my son's killers; I did not wish them dead; I did not wish them in jail. If I had to, I could take their children and raise them as my own." In the face of unspeakable violation and heartbreak, she refused to be shamed into silence and isolation. She refused to bear the shame of a shameless culture. She enveloped herself in community, and in so doing gathered the courage to expand her practice of community to larger and larger circles–to the extent of including her son's acquitted killers.

Under conditions of extreme domination and the threat of death, people throughout the ages have found ways to embrace an alternative model of power. Consider, for example, the mothers of the disappeared in Latin America. These are the women who met in dark churches, refusing to submit to the isolation imposed by a violent, oppressive, militaristic regime. These are the women who marched silently in public plazas wearing the names of their disappeared children embroidered on their shawls. Their strategies exemplify one version of alternative practice called "defecting in place." Coined by Kathleen Fischer (1999), defecting in place is both a strategy and a metaphor signifying a departure from the old ways of thinking and relating, while being present in a whole new way. It is occupying a space within the parameters of the old structure and filling it with alternative community. Like the mothers of the disappeared, women who defect in place stay connected to their feeling-thoughts, and thereby increase the possibilities for connection with others. They come together to experience and refine an alternative power, one that is much closer to love.

To embrace an alternative power is to relinquish any fantasies of happy endings. The status quo works ceaselessly through a variety of means to perpetuate itself, and it does not tolerate disruption well. Ours is a culture that codifies identities, rank orders those identities by worth, and dispenses prizes–both real and illusory–based on compliance with the designated roles. It should come as no surprise then that opposition to alternative power comes in many faces, shapes, and genders. We often fail to recognize the operation of dominating, deterministic power because it carries the faces of those nearest to our hearts. It sometimes bears faces that look much like our own. In other words, in subverting the dominant patriarchal paradigm, the adversary we encounter is not always the adversary we expect. It is often the case that the persons most opposed to an alternative paradigm are the very persons who are subjugated in power-over systems. Such reactivity is predictable when understood as an expression of the relational paradox. Safety seems to reside in the illusion of connection, in not risking conflict that might upend the ordered arrangements of the status quo, particularly when those arrangements provide a modicum of privilege over and against others.

Envisioning an alternative paradigm of power often results in having to leave unyielding relationships. When it is clear that a disconnection is intractable, the only reasonable response may be to leave the relationship. To quote Rubin (1998):

> When you have tried everything, and your opponent remains an adversary, walk away. It is the only way to keep your spiritual and emotional initiative for another day.

Chronic, deadening disconnection is characterized by a perpetual lack of mutuality. There is no possibility for growth-enhancing connection or mutual empowerment. Under those conditions, to walk away is to make a bold claim on renewal and relational possibility.

For much of my inspiration, I rely on the tradition of song. In American black tradition there is a spiritual entitled "Go Down, Moses." "Go down, Moses. Tell Old Pharaoh to let my people go . . ." Tell Old Pharaoh to free the enslaved, the oppressed. In speaking to conditions of 20th and 21st century enslavement, singer Roberta Flack (1971) exhorted the oppressed to let Pharaoh go. In her song "Go Up, Moses," Flack offered a brilliant insight into the manipulative dependency of dominating power. She sang that Pharaoh doesn't want or value you, but he needs you. Without you, there is no Pharaoh.

Faced with the manipulative dependencies and the false prizes of the power-over paradigm, the greatest challenge is at times to let Pharaoh go. To let Pharaoh go is to take responsibility for examining the degree to which we have internalized the values of the power-over paradigm, creating an inclination to dominate and control others. To let Pharaoh go is to claim our competencies, to nurture our capacities, and to embrace accountability to a new paradigm of power in relationship.

REFERENCES

Brock, R. N. (1993). Journeys by heart: A christology of erotic power. New York: Crossroads Press.

Dorn, J., Flack, R., & Jackson, J. (1971). Go Up, Moses. [Recorded by Flack, R.]. On Quiet Fire [CD]. New York: Atlantic Records.

Fischer, K. (1999). Transforming fire: Women using anger creatively. Mahwah, NJ: Paulist Press.
Fletcher, J., Jordan, J., & Miller, J. (2000). Women and the workplace: Applications of psychodynamic theory. The American Journal of Psychoanalysis, 60(3), 243-261.
hooks, b. (2000). Feminist theory: From margin to center (2nd ed.). Cambridge, MA: South End Press.
Janeway, E. (1980). Powers of the weak. New York: Knopf.
Jordan, J. V. (1991). Empathy and self boundaries. In J. Jordan, A. Kaplan, J. Miller, I. Stiver, & J. Surrey (Eds.). Women's growth in connection. New York: Guilford Press.
Jordan, J. V. (2002, April). Courage in connection: Working with vulnerability. Paper presented at the Harvard Learning from Women Conference co-sponsored by Harvard Medical School/Cambridge Hospital and the Jean Baker Miller Training Institute, Boston, MA.
Kollias, K. (1975). Class realities: Creating a new power base. Quest, 1(3), 28-43.
Miller, J. B. (1986). Toward a new psychology of women (2nd ed.). Boston: Beacon Press.
Miller, J. B. (1991). Women and power. In J. Jordan, A. Kaplan, J. Miller, I. Stiver, & J. Surrey (Eds.). Women's growth in connection. New York: Guilford Press.
Rubin, H. (1998). The princessa: Machiavelli for women. New York: Dell Books.
Stiver, I. (1991). Work inhibitions in women. In J. Jordan, A. Kaplan, J. Miller, I. Stiver, & J. Surrey (Eds.). Women's growth in connection. New York: Guilford Press.
Thomas, D. (2002). Unpublished symposium comments. Harvard University, February 6, 2002.
Walker, A. (1979). Janie Crawford in Good night, Willie Lee, I'll See You in the Morning. San Diego: Harvest/Harcourt Brace and Janovich.
Williamson, M. (1996). A return to love: Reflections on the principles of a course in miracles. New York: HarperCollins.

Telling the Truth About Power

Jean Baker Miller

SUMMARY. In this culture, those in power do not usually talk about it and the rest of us tend not to recognize it either. A similar situation exists in therapy, where the therapist herself may not be aware of her own power-over tactics. This article suggests methods that may help therapists to acknowledge their power and also to change from power-over actions to mutually empowering relationships. From this line of thinking, there follows an exploration of altering the concept of boundaries in therapy into mutually constructed agreements between patient and therapist. This article was presented at the Summer Training Institute of the Jean Baker Miller Training Institute, June, 2003.

Jean Baker Miller MD (1927-2006), was Founding Scholar and Director of the Jean Baker Miller Training Institute at the Stone Center, Wellesley College; Clinical Professor of Psychiatry at Boston University School of Medicine; author of *Toward a New Psychology of Women*; and co-author of *The Healing Connection: How Women Form Relationships in Therapy and in Life*, and *Women's Growth in Connection*.

HIDDEN POWER

They tell women not to begin by apologizing, but after working on this talk, I do think I have to amend the title to "Telling Some Truth About Some Kinds of Power." You'll see why.

Many of us in this society (and in some others too) are mixed up about power. Yet power is very real and is operating right in front of us all the time. Quite amazingly, those who have the most power in our society almost never talk about it and even more amazingly induce many of the rest of us not to recognize it either.

As an example, when I was a kid, my friends and I adored going to the movies. We'd go every Saturday afternoon, and for five cents we'd always see two full-length films, a cartoon, a newsreel, and an episode, or what we called a "chapter," of some long ongoing adventure story, which was almost always a Western. Every week we'd see the "bad guys," the so-called Indians, portrayed as strange-looking, fierce, uncivilized, savage murderers who were threatening the White cowboys. While I must say that we girls did not join in, the theater rang with ear shattering cries, cheers, whoops, and whistles when the cowboys hurt or killed the Native Americans.

It never occurred to us that it was the White people who had taken power by force, robbing the Native Americans' land and destroying their cultures, even calling them by a false name. We absorbed these untruths routinely every week. Thus, you can see how I was drawn into disparaging and even fearing these powerful, violent people (from where I lived in the heart of New York City). I don't remember history classes in elementary or high school changing these images, and I can't recall how old I was before I was shocked to learn the truth that we, Whites, had brutally taken power over the Native Americans. Likewise, we never saw any other people of color portrayed with any truth. This is an easy example of how the "cultural materials" of a dominant group mystify its operation of power. While everyone may fail to recognize this power-over situation, those closest to the dominant group may be the most likely to do so, e.g., White, middle- or upper-class women.

Is it not similar in therapy? Clearly, the therapist has a huge amount of power over the patient but traditionally has not talked about it. Alfred Adler drew attention to the topic of power early in the history of the psychoanalytic movement, but he was cast out by Freud, and little was heard about it after that. It was really the feminist therapy movement and the movement by therapists of marginalized groups that opened up this whole topic only fairly recently. It makes sense that this was the case.

A group that becomes dominant in any society tends to divide people with less power into groups for various historical reasons. These less powerful groups can include divisions by race, class, gender, sexual preference, and the like. The dominant group often gains tremendous power over the less powerful groups in all realms, including economic, social, political, and cultural. But dominant groups do not usually say, "I have great power over your life; I want to keep it and if possible, increase it because I'm afraid of losing any of it to you."

Now, here comes a tedious part. Along with the obscurity surrounding power comes confusion in the usage of the word. Without reviewing everyone else's definitions, let me say that we have used the phrase "power-to" to mean the ability to make a change in any situation, large or small, i.e., the ability to move anything from point A to point B without the connotation of restricting or forcing anyone else. For the later forms of power that imply force, we've used the term, "power-over."

In a basic sense, power-over usually follows from the structural situation whereby one group has more resources and privilege and thus, has more capacity to force or control others. This is the structural power I just referred to above.

Structural power is most influential and most important to recognize. However, in a complicated society there may be variations within, for example today, when an African American woman supervisor may have some power over a White male worker, this usually exists only in the workplace and not when they step outside. Also, even if a dominant group has overwhelming amounts of power over subordinates, subordinates often find some means of exerting power. These can be power-over attempts or power-to actions. For example, in the play, *The Servant*, British playwright Harold Pinter portrays a clever "man servant" gradually gaining total power over his master. The master is an aristocrat who is reduced to complete dependence because he has been so advantaged that he has not learned how to operate in the world. Such an example, however, does not change the situation of structural power in the world.

At times, subordinates can find the power to resist the force of the dominant group and also add to their power to move toward some structural change, as in the example of Rosa Parks, who began by resisting the insult of bus segregation. That act became a major step in the civil rights movement. What's more, although history books often lead us to believe that resistance to the dominant group is principally achieved through the separate acts of heroic individuals, this, as in the case of Rosa Parks, is a simplistic understanding. It is important to note that

Rosa Parks was not alone in her efforts, but was working with others in her community as a long-time active member of the NAACP.

Rethinking conceptualizations of power, Judith Jordan (1986) and Jan Surrey (1987) have developed the concept of *mutual empowerment.* This is different from the idea of empowerment and is a complicated concept. I think we can most readily understand it in an example I will use below; so I'll hold it until then. So much for definitions for now, but it's even more complex with the many intricacies to be explained at another time.

Clearly, the members of subordinate groups could benefit by joining together within each group and across groups to create change in their conditions. However, in addition to material force, dominant groups usually manufacture false belief systems that act to keep them apart. These belief systems operate in many ways.

PREVENTING CHANGE

For one thing, dominant groups tend to protect the advantages, rewards, and spoils of disconnection by erecting barriers to change. They usually create a whole social structure and culture based on fear–fear of economic suffering, social ostracism, political deprivation, and more. It becomes more complex if we add psychological dimensions. Patricia Hill Collins, an African American sociologist, gives us a basis for understanding these dimensions (1990). In prior work, we have discussed her concept of *controlling images* (CIs). Dominant groups tend to create sets of images about themselves and each of the "subordinate" groups, e.g., those savage Native Americans, the "Black Mammy," the "China doll," and the like. As Collins says, these images are always false but exert a powerful influence and act to hold each group in its place, that is, they act against change. We all absorb these images about others and ourselves, usually without fully realizing it, as in the example of the Native Americans above. Thus, we think we know (usually wrongly) what it would be like to be a member of any of the groups other than our own. Both dominants and subordinates are thereby held in place.

For dominants, the great threat is to be reduced to being like one or more of the subordinate groups. Peggy McIntosh (1995), a White writer brought up in the upper-middle-class, wrote that she now realizes her whole upbringing was really based on the premise that if she didn't behave properly, that is, live up to the CIs for her class and race, she would become like one of those "lesser people." So those closest to the dominant group live with the threat that one can always be cast out of the group of the "desirables."

For subordinates, there are always the threats of direct loss of the small amount of status or resources they may have, even if they are scant. For example, White women were often made to feel they would not be real women if they did not adhere to the stereotypes of a "proper woman"–a heterosexual good mother. They would lose the advantages they gain by being linked to White men. In a different situation, such as in the novel, *The Women of Brewster Place*, Gloria Naylor (1983) portrays a young African American activist woman, Kiswana Brown, who is trying to organize a neighborhood of poor Black women. Her mother, Mrs. Brown, a woman who has become middle class, comes to warn her that she should stop this work now that she could have more in life. Thus, power-over societies mystify their practices to entice many of us, all the less powerful, into cooperation with them, as Maureen Walker has said (2000c).

HIDDEN POWER IN THERAPY

Clearly, therapists have more power than patients. We and others, especially feminist therapists and therapists from marginalized groups, have discussed this in prior writings (see for example Brown, 1994; Lerman & Porter, 1990; Comas-Diaz & Greene, 1994; Pinderhughes, 1989; Veldhuis, 2001). I won't review all of the valuable writing here but will mention a few examples of the points they've made. For example, the patient is asked to reveal a great deal about her most intimate, painful or shameful thoughts, feelings, and behaviors. She is therefore in a much more exposed and vulnerable position. She is presumed to be the "sick" person while the therapist is presumed to be "healthy" and psychologically mature. The therapist is assumed to be the expert; thus she is in command of the discourse. If the therapist is from a class or racial group that has more status in society, this will add to the power differential and the patient's difficulty in addressing it.

Sometimes, most powerful of all, the patient cares more about the therapist than the therapist does about her. She knows that the therapist is at the center of her life but assumes she is only one of many to the therapist (Eldridge, Mencher, & Slater, 1997). Feminist therapists, for example, Laura Brown (1994), Hannah Lerman and Natalie Porter (1990), and more recently Cindy Veldhuis (2001) have described many other ways–verbal, nonverbal, obvious, and subtle–in which this power is reinforced. They have emphasized that therapists may fail to recognize their power and act in "power-over" ways without realizing it. They believe that this may be the most destructive use of power.

Because of the history of often feeling powerless or even because of their egalitarian ideology, White women therapists may have a particular tendency to deny their power. For example, Cindy Veldhuis (2001) wrote:

> Therapists who fail to recognize their own place of increased power in the relationship in effect negate a client's reality (Brown, 1994). Clients typically see us as having some structural or symbolic power, and when we deny that, we deny their reality, and are at risk for losing our ability to understand the relationship from their perspective. When we are aware of our power, we are consciously aware of how our actions, or inactions, affect the client. We recognize that even a brief discontinuation of eye contact may signal something profound to the client. . . . If that eye contact flickers, and we see the impact in the client's face, we can use our power to attend to the moment, and discuss what happened. In doing so, we introduce a new power into the relationship, the power of mutual respect. (Siegel & Lawson, 1990, p. 53)

I think this is a most cogent short summary of the idea, but we have to note that holding eye contact is not something that is done in all cultures.

Thus, like members of the dominant group, therapists can deny our power and act to prevent change in therapy. Last year, at this Institute, we explored the ways in which we as therapists can turn to power-over maneuvers rather than toward connection, especially when we, ourselves, feel inadequate, anxious, exposed, shamed, or similar difficult feelings (Miller, 2002). I want to explore some more of the hidden ways in which we use power-over maneuvers in therapy that prevent change.

As an example we can use the video that Judy Jordan role-played (1998); I think many here have seen it. If not, you can probably follow the idea. In it, the patient, Martha, becomes angry and quite insulting to Judy. Judy could have said something like what therapists often say, "I see you're angry. I was just trying to give you a helpful suggestion." Instead, Judy says that she sees how she may have sounded like the patient's unhelpful family members and friends. Thus, she acknowledges that there may be reasons for Martha's anger when seen within Martha's experience. Judy importantly adds that she, Judy, may have been unhelpful in what she said and tells the patient that she feels bad about that.

After a few more exchanges, Martha and Judy become more responsive and more connected.

Here we see an example of how a therapist could easily have used the power of presumed expertise to make a patient feel even more irrational, angry, confused, or sicker. Judy could have been even subtler in her power-over response, e.g., asking the patient to explore her anger further. Depending on how it is done, such a question can convey that there is something wrong or unhealthy that should be examined. In any case, it may not be the best step toward building connection *at that moment*. By contrast, Judy uses her truly valuable expertise, that is, her empathy, authenticity, openness, and trying to move toward connection. She demonstrates that she has heard Martha, and as a result, Martha sees she has had an impact and thus feels more power in the relationship.

All this brings up the question of the goals of therapy. I would suggest that the first goal is that patient and therapist feel more connected through the patient feeling that the therapist is empathic, understanding, and responsive. This is essential for the work of therapy.

Second, if the patient feels more connected, she becomes more able to explore painful and difficult feelings. The therapist grows as well, but not at the expense of the patient. Rather, she has *participated* in moving toward more connection and toward the patient's increase in power and growth. This participation always adds to the therapist's growth. All of this is to say that both people and the relationship, as in the example with Martha, have moved toward more effectiveness and power–what we have called mutual empowerment, not one person up and one down.

Here again, I think I need to review some definitions. There is great confusion around our use of the term "mutual empowerment." In all relationships such as parent-child, teacher-student, therapist-patient, and the like, one person clearly has more power than the other; they are not the same, nor are they equal along various dimensions, e.g., age, experience, knowledge of a certain field, etc. Note–these forms of unequal relationships are not the same as the inequalities forced upon certain social groups. In unequal relationships like parent-child, teacher-student, and therapist-patient relationships the goal is for the more powerful person to foster the growth of the other person, that is, to move *toward* change and toward equality (Miller, 1976). This movement may take a long time as it does in the parent-child relationship.

Even without equality there can be mutuality and movement toward more mutuality, as we use the term. Mutuality means joining together in a kind of relationality in which both (or all) participants are engaged, empathic, and growing (Jordan, 1986). Martha and Judy offer an example.

Likewise, a parent and child and also the people in other unequal relationships may participate in many moments when they join in mutual engagement that is benefiting them both, though usually not in the same way or on the same level. We can see this even in studies of mother-infant interaction, e.g., in Tronick's (1998) and others' work. Obviously the two people are not the same, nor are they equal.

Most importantly, in the therapist-client, the parent-child, and other similarly constructed unequal relationships the more powerful person must take primary responsibility for developing the relationship. The more powerful person has to keep trying to find ways to make the interactions growth fostering, i.e., moving toward fuller mutuality–and eventually equality. We don't know fully how to do this in any of these unequal relationships, including therapy, but we see it as our task to continue this search. I do believe that one central problem is that we carry over the ways of behaving that we've learned from the power-over structure of our society, again, often without recognizing it (Miller, 1976).

SOME PRACTICAL STEPS IN THERAPY

In a previous paper we've described what we've called "creative moments in therapy" (Stiver, Rosen, Surrey, & Miller, 2000). These are moments when the patient presents us with a difficult dilemma and we are forced out of our usual comfort zone and into thinking and doing something new. These steps often make us feel vulnerable, at risk, and as if we are stretching ourselves psychologically. As a result, we often found we've moved into better connection, a bit like the episode in Judy's video mentioned earlier. I wonder if we can explore some specific steps or guides that we might build into therapy that would increase the patient's power and challenge us to recognize our own power all along in therapy? These guides would make working with power dynamics a recognized central part of what we do in therapy all the time, rather than something we do in response to crises. The power of the therapist is so much greater than the patient's that perhaps it is important to create some standard overt safeguards and guides for ourselves. We've talked about mutual empowerment, but we need to delineate better how to actually bring it about.

Joyce Fletcher (1999) has described a similar process in the workplace, calling it "fluid expertise." This process explains how both employees and supervisors have something to contribute, and that these contributions can pass back and forth between them rather than being fixed in one person. This interaction increases the employee's power in the workplace. In addition, in this form of interaction, two or more people can create something new, more than either one would be able to create alone. They also find a new kind of relational experience, the experience that comes when two or more people engage together and find the vigor of this kind of connection, what I'd call the *five good things* that come with this mutual experience (Miller, 1988; Miller & Stiver, 1997).

Can we find specific ways that would encourage movement toward greater mutual empowerment in therapy? Last year we began such a list (Miller, 2002), and today perhaps we can add a few more. For example, can we begin at the first session? We all try to explain to clients how we work in therapy and gear the session to the specific person. For example, I could say something along the lines of an introduction to my approach to therapy that stresses the mutual nature of the experience: "What we do is talk together and try to find out what's making you feel anxious, depressed, etc., and how we can change that. This may sound different from other kinds of treatment you've had, but it's important that you try to say what you think and feel. I will respond as honestly as I can. From this back and forth we often discover what will help. So what you say is really important." We then have to talk about time, money, and the like; I will add more about that below. For people from cultures that have a very different expectation about treatment, the therapist has to discuss much more about this form of therapy and also make more adaptations to cultural beliefs.

Would it be possible to add some thoughts that may help the patient feel more power in the relationship, such as, "If I say anything that you don't understand, please tell me"? Or, "If I say anything you don't like, it would be very good if you can let me know. This will help our work." Or, "If I say anything that bothers you in other ways, it's important that you say so." Here, again, such questions may be too different from the expectations of people from some cultures and the therapist will have to adapt accordingly.

Other questions might include, "What is your greatest fear? What is your greatest fear in the outside world? Here in therapy? What is your greatest wish? In the outer world? In here? If patient and therapist are from different class, cultural, or other backgrounds, or have different sexual preferences, such questions may lead into talking about these differences. If they don't, therapists can raise their thoughts and questions about these differences either in the first session or as soon as they feel they are appropriate. As therapy proceeds, therapists should continue to discuss these differences, for in this society, they always contain issues of power. We are stressing how all patients experience the therapist as so much more powerful; this differential can be much greater if the patient has been made to feel less worthy and powerful because of the societal CIs forced upon her.

I'm certain that all of you can think of more and better questions. More important than their specific value, these questions may convey a general *attitude* that invites the patient to take more power in the relationship. In addition, we can ask ourselves all along in the course of therapy if and how our power is operating in some power-over way, especially but not only when therapy may not be moving well. We can ask the patient directly if she is feeling some effects of this power. But it may not be clear to her or she may not feel able to answer, so we have to work at finding out together. Obviously, such questions would have to be geared to each individual person, but we could develop an overall framework that we then use in future cases.

BOUNDARIES

This discussion may have led some of you to think about boundaries. I would like to explore the question of boundaries as another example of the ways we may use them (or something like them) to increase the patient's power. I believe that the traditional concept of boundaries can be another example of obscuring power in therapy.

Again, feminist therapists (see, for example, Brown, 1994) and members of the JBMTI have discussed several valuable ways of exploring the concept. For example, Judy Jordan has described boundaries as really about clarity and most of all about boundaries as places of meeting rather than separation (Jordan, 1995; Jordan & Hartling, 2002; Miller et al., 1999). She has explored several ways of examining them, especially illuminating the ways therapists may use boundaries to obscure their use of power, that is, ways that really protect themselves rather than serve the patient. But patients violate boundaries too or at least we say they do. I will address that issue.

Further, the concept of feminist ethics is closely related to the topic of boundaries. Along with other feminist therapists, we have discussed framing the ethics of therapy in a positive way rather than as a set of prohibitions (Brown, 1994; Lerman & Porter, 1990). I believe a positive approach can be translated into the question: *how do we build mutually empowering connections that lead to healing and growth?*

Usually the therapist decides what a boundary is and what a violation of it is. Is it possible for this to become a more mutual process? I believe so, but want to repeat that the therapist always has the responsibility of making this and all parts of the relationship growth-fostering.

THE UNDERLYING BASIS OF "BOUNDARIES"

Any concept of boundaries rests on an underlying theory of therapy and of development and growth. A central tenet of RCT is the *Central Relational Paradox* (CRP), which is the idea that people yearn for connection and also fear it or parts of it because they have had hurtful, frightening, humiliating, or sometimes terrifying relationship experiences in the past (Miller, 1988; Miller & Stiver, 1997). People who have suffered trauma or severe psychological isolation may fear it most intensely, but we all do to various degrees. As a result, we continue to try to find connections though we also develop *strategies of disconnection* (SDs; Miller & Stiver, 1997). These are the psychological strategies we use to keep parts of ourselves out of connection, the parts that we have come to believe are unacceptable. Many, not all, so-called boundary violations are reflections of the CRP and are analogous to SDs. They are attempts to maintain connection in the only way a person can find in the midst of great fear.

The therapy situation especially lends itself to this kind of fear and confusion because, in addition to the other reasons for feeling the therapist's great power, the patient may begin to feel some possibly deeper, more true connection. Then she begins to fear that this openness to connection will lead to the kind of harm that occurred when she was open to connection in her prior experience. She may also fear that her SDs, which she desperately believes are so essential, are at risk, i.e., the powerful pull toward connection is now so much stronger yet she so fears losing what seem like her only protections. She tries to do the only things she can in the face of this intense dilemma.

At such times, people's actions usually grow out of the confusion about what connection can lead to. People are usually not aware of or at all clear about this complicated mixture of feelings. For example, in another paper, Judy Jordan (2003) described a patient who told everyone in the hospital about Judy's so-called "mistakes" and "bad treatment." It eventually became clear that this patient deeply yearned to connect with

Judy, but she was simultaneously using a strategy to protect herself from the imagined dangers of being alone with Judy by publicly criticizing Judy's work. Not surprisingly, this woman had been severely and secretly abused as a child.

I had a patient who soon into therapy, began to phone me repeatedly after every session feeling very disorganized, panicked, and sometimes suicidal. It seemed that our meetings made her worse! Much later we were able to clarify that her father, a man with serious and chronic illness, often acted in a seemingly interested and loving way but sometimes also terrified her with the accusation that she made him feel tired and sicker. Later in her childhood he died. As she moved into connection and began to feel that I had real interest and concern for her, she equated those feelings with the confused expectation that she would make me sick and weak. This meant that I would then abandon her. I think she may also have felt angry that I now seemed to have so much power over her. Thus, the possibility of connection can create a sense of vulnerability for all of us and we may not be at all clear about this. For some people it can be extremely confusing and frightening.

SDs often contain an aspect of coercion because they can be attempts to use power-over tactics, which are then called boundary violations. These strategies may be the only source of power the patient can find in her confusion and fear. They are also power maneuvers in the sense that they interfere with the forward movement of therapy because this movement can seem as if it is leading to such dire consequences. This is really saying that they are attempts to use power-over actions to counter what feels like the threat that the therapist's power will be like the power-over actions in her past.

EXPLORING ALTERNATIVES

What is the answer? I think it is to try to find the ways that the patient can find legitimate power to face this threat. She will then not need coercion for protection. This will not work all at once, but perhaps if we think of it this way, we can work toward this empowerment.

How to do this? Can we think in terms of "agreements" rather then boundaries? (I don't want to suggest new words now but perhaps we should eventually do so. I think the word "boundaries" is misleading and comes out of one kind of theoretical thinking. At the beginning of therapy, patient and therapist can set up their agreements about their work together. These could include, for example:

- The therapist can explain how she works, including the things we usually say about the framework of therapy as mentioned above, e.g., confidentiality, time arrangements, money, cancellation policy, and the like. She can ask the patient if she can agree with these arrangements. Are there some different arrangements she'd prefer? If the therapist can't agree to the patient's requests, she should say so and explain why. As Judy Jordan (Miller et al., 1998) has suggested, the therapist should say if her reasons are based on her knowledge in the field or even just her own personal desires or limits, and not that the patient has asked for something excessive. One way of fulfilling this approach would be for the therapist to say that she believes meeting only every two weeks will not be enough to help or that the therapist can't make evening sessions because of her other obligations.
- The therapist should say that agreements can be altered by joint discussion as therapy proceeds. This would put these changes in the realm of discussion rather than some sacred mandates. It would indicate that the patient can have an effect on the relationship.
- The therapist should include here all of the things she will not do that would harm the patient, e.g., violate confidentiality, engage in other relationships with the patient outside of therapy, engage in sexual relations with the patient, etc. I think this is still important to say very concretely.
- Later, if violations occur, these agreements can be referred to. Again, we can help the patient explore whether she feels that some change in the arrangements can help rather than make the patient feel she has violated some sacred rules. Of course, the patient may still feel compelled to try to violate the agreements in a non-direct way, but at least she has more of a chance to move toward more direct power.

It will often be possible to make some change in the agreements that can begin to allay the patient's fears if we stay open to hearing them. For example, regarding the illustration above of the patient who phoned me repeatedly after every session, the patient and I made an agreement that she would phone once at a set time after each appointment. If that did not feel to be enough, she would leave messages after the first call; we agreed that I would not return those calls unless she specifically requested it.

She felt she could legitimately ask to talk with me at those times, rather than feeling she was always wrong to call and yet calling repeatedly. She almost never requested more than the one call; this agreement seemed to be enough, as it is for some people. Also, it may have relieved her fears that she was hurting and weakening me. Often just the discussion of these issues within connection can afford some relief. It can open up some of the whole realm of terror and isolation in which they are encased. In this instance we made this new agreement long before we understood exactly what lay behind this woman's great fears.

Incidentally, this vignette offers an illustration of the ways in which the theory of therapy can guide us to constructive or destructive ways of working. In traditional terms, this patient could have been seen as "very demanding" (based on orality, dependence, etc.). As Irene Stiver used to say, such formulations do not give you much help in discovering what to do (1984).

As indicated above, patients often cannot tell at these times what they are feeling and why. If that is the case, at least the therapist is conveying that there's a reason for her feelings, whatever they are. This can contrast with many discussions about boundaries that make patients feel even more irrational, disturbed, ashamed, guilty, and often angry with the therapist for making her have all these dreadful feelings.

Even before patient and therapist fully understand the issue, they can often find some interim way of trying to deal with the difficulties, such as with the phone call plan in the illustration above. If this plan isn't working, perhaps together they can come up with other attempts, e.g., rather than immediately phoning, a patient might try writing for three minutes about what she feels like doing or what she wishes from the therapist, or the like. The act of writing may lead her into some understanding of a workable plan. In any case, such a discussion about alternatives can demonstrate that the therapist wants to keep trying to find the ways to increase the patient's power.

Along with these efforts, the therapist can keep examining whether she is using power in a way she herself may not recognize. Sometimes power-over strategies may arise from the therapeutic CIs, that is, therapists' notions about the images they must uphold, as discussed in prior papers (Walker, 2002b).

Thus, a seeming paradox, but not really–the way to prevent or reduce what are called patients' boundary violations is to work to increase the patient's power in the relationship but power-in-connection rather than power that is coercive arising out of fear. I believe this discussion illustrates the point Jordan made that the concept of boundaries is anchored in a model of separation (Jordan, 1995). By contrast, I am suggesting a concept based on a model of connection. So, in summary, perhaps we can change the concept of boundaries into a joint endeavor that patient and therapist develop together, rather than one in which the therapist is laying down laws. Even the attempt to do so may keep therapists focused on questions of power and help us to overcome our own denial and mystification.

CONCLUSION

Because we live in a culture that operates on a power-over basis and also tends to obscure the use of power, we are very likely to act in these ways ourselves in therapy, especially in times of difficulty, feelings of inadequacy, shame, or fear. As Maureen Walker has said, this is so likely to be our "default position" (Walker, 2002c). So our constant endeavor must be to seek the ways we, as therapists, are acting that are not mutually empowering, especially when we may not be aware of these, and most especially, because they may be culturally syntonic and "therapeutic culture syntonic."

I believe we need ongoing education on this issue and we need to create more specific "forms," or ways of thinking and acting that will help us to see what we may not be seeing. The issue of power may constitute another reason why we should all continue in ongoing peer or supervision groups because alone, we cannot easily become aware of what we're not aware of. We all need other people's input. Peer groups could add the stated goal of doing this inquiry about power for each other.

In saying all this, we are really talking about trying to work beyond the values of our society, that is, when we talk about bringing authenticity, mutual empathy, and mutual empowerment to the relationship. Even in its origins therapy was seen as unearthing aspects of life that society kept hidden. With Freud it was sex. Later therapists found it was not sex alone but a whole context of relationships, although these were initially discussed in terms derived from sex and drive theories, such as oral or dependency needs. Today, perhaps more basic than all, we are beginning to recognize the forms of power by which one group of people keeps others from full development and seduces us all to cooperate and collude in doing so both on the larger social scene and also in our most intimate relationships—even in therapy, the setting in which we are trying to be healers.

It is not that the patient's greater power will mean less power for the therapist. As we've said, that kind of thinking usually follows from a notion of a "zero-sum game." It follows from patriarchal, power-over thinking. Instead, it is a question of reframing the issue altogether in different terms.

The answer is not to just flip over whoever is in the position of power so that the subordinates gain more power but continue operating in the same old dominant-subordinate framework. The issue is to create a new structure altogether. I think we can see this quite clearly in therapy. The goal is to enter into connections that facilitate the patient's growth. As the patient grows, she does not gain more "power-over" but power to enter into better and deeper connection, the most valuable power of all. We have to keep trying to find more and better ways to do this. As we do so, we do not become less powerful, but more powerful in terms of our knowledge, our capacities, and the growth that comes from participating in growth-fostering connection.

Because we work at this intersection where change and growth occur, perhaps we can illuminate further the ways to do this on the larger scene, where they are so sorely needed. Certainly, we pursue similar goals in child rearing, teaching, and the like. But maybe we can contribute on an even broader scale in public life.

Perhaps we can help to find the ways whereby less powerful groups of people can not only gain power but recast the operation of power, transform the very nature of power. This transformation would change life for all of us.

REFERENCES

Brown, L. S. (1994). *Subversive dialogues.* New York: Basic Books.
Collins, P. H. (1990). *Black feminist thought.* New York: Routledge.
Comas-Diaz, L., & Greene, B. (1994). *Women of color.* New York: Guilford Press.
Eldridge, N., Mencher, J., & Slater, S. (1993). The conundrum of mutuality: a lesbian dialogue. *Work in Progress, No. 62.* Wellesley, MA: Stone Center Working Paper Series.
Feminist Therapy Institute. (1990). Feminist Therapy Institute code of ethics. In H. Lerman & N. Porter (Eds.). Feminist ethics in psychotherapy. New York: Springer.
Fletcher, J. (1999). *Disappearing acts: Gender, power, and relational practice at work.* Cambridge, MA: MIT Press.
Jordan, J. V. (1986). The meaning of mutuality. *Work in Progress, No. 23.* Wellesley, MA: Stone Center Working Paper Series.

Jordan, J. V. (1995). Boundaries: A relational perspective. *Psychotherapy Forum, 1*(2), 4-5.
Jordan, J. V. (1998). Clinical Vignettes: "Martha." [Videotape, No. 5]. Wellesley, MA: Stone Center Working Paper Series.
Jordan, J. V. (2003). Valuing vulnerability: New models of courage. *Work in Progress, No. 102.* Wellesley, MA: Stone Center Working Paper Series.
Jordan, J. V., & Hartling, L. M. (2002). New developments in Relational-Cultural Theory. In M. Ballou & L. S. Brown, (Eds.). *Rethinking mental health and disorder: Feminist perspectives.* New York: Guilford Press.
Lerman, H., & Porter, N. (Eds.). (1990). *Feminist ethics in psychotherapy.* New York: Springer.
McIntosh, P. (2000). Feeling like a fraud, Part III. *Work in Progress, No. 90.* Wellesley, MA: Stone Center Working Paper Series.
Miller, J. B. (1976). *Toward a new psychology of women.* Boston: Beacon Press.
Miller, J. B. (1988). Connections, disconnections, and violations. *Work in Progress, No. 33.* Wellesley, MA: Stone Center Working Paper Series.
Miller, J. B. (2002). How change happens: controlling images, mutuality, and power. *Work in Progress, No. 96.* Wellesley, MA: Stone Center Working Paper Series.
Miller, J. B., & Stiver, I. P. (1997). *The healing connection.* Boston: Beacon Press.
Miller, J. B., Jordan, J. V., Stiver, I. P., Walker, M., Surrey, J., & Eldridge, N. (1999). Therapists' authenticity. *Work in Progress, No. 82.* Wellesley, MA: Stone Center Working Paper Series.
Naylor, G. (1983). *The women of Brewster Place.* New York: Penguin Books.
Pinderhughes, E. (1989*). Understanding race, ethnicity, and power: Key to efficacy in clinical practice.* New York: Free Press.
Siegel, R. J., & Larsin, C. (1990). The ethics of power differentials. In H. Lerman & N. Porter (Eds.). *Feminist ethics in psychotherapy.* New York: Springer.
Stiver, I. P. (1984). Personal Communication.
Stiver, I. P., Rosen, W., Surrey, J., & Miller, J. B. (2000). Creative moments in Relational-Cultural Therapy. *Work in Progress, No. 92.* Wellesley: MA: Stone Center Working Paper Series.
Surrey, J. (1987). Relationship and empowerment. *Work in Progress, No. 30.* Wellesley, MA: Stone Center Working Paper Series.
Tronick, E. (1998). Dyadically expanded states of consciousness and the process of therapeutic change. *Infant Mental Health Journal, 19*(3), 290-299.
Veldhuis, C. (2001). The trouble with power. In E. Kaschak (Ed.). *The next generation: Third wave feminist psychotherapy.* New York: The Haworth Press.
Walker, M. (2002a). Power and effectiveness: Envisioning an alternate paradigm. *Work in Progress, No. 94.* Wellesley, MA: Stone Center Working Paper Series.
Walker, M. (2002b). How therapy helps when the culture hurts. *Work in Progress, No. 95.* Wellesley, MA: Stone Center Working Paper Series.
Walker, M. (2002c). Personal Communication.

SECTION THREE: RCT AND SOCIAL JUSTICE

Introduction to Section Three: RCT and Social Justice

In the third and final section the writers focus on the social application of relational-cultural work: how does RCT help us better understand organizational and social phenomena and support social justice? In the first article in this section, Hartling and Sparks outline the difficulties when practitioners who may use relational-cultural practices in their work find themselves in non-relational, disconnected work contexts. In "Learning at the Margin: New Models of Strength," Jordan looks at the ways in which marginalization, the use of power-over maneuvers and privilege contribute to disconnection at a personal and societal level. Strength in vulnerability is proposed as an alternative to strength in isolation. She continues this theme in the next article, "Valuing Vulnerability: New Definitions of Courage," as she challenges the illusion of an invulnerable and separate self, which is espoused by the dominant culture. And in "Commitment to Connection in a Culture of Fear," Jordan examines the ways in which cultural and personal denial of fear and vulnerability contribute to a sense of isolation. She looks at how fear is manipulated in hierarchical settings to ensure the preservation of existing power arrangements.

Relational-Cultural Practice: Working in a Nonrelational World

Linda Hartling
Elizabeth Sparks

SUMMARY. While more and more clinicians are practicing a relational-cultural approach to therapy, many work in settings that continue to reinforce the normative values of separation and disconnection. Consequently, practitioners face the challenges of helping clients heal and grow-through-connection while navigating work settings that are all too often professionally disempowering, disconnecting, and isolating, i.e., "cultures of disconnection." This article begins a conversation about the complexities of practicing Relational-Cultural Theory in nonrelational work situations and explores new possibilities for creating movement and change in these settings.

Linda M. Hartling, PhD, is Associate Director, Jean Baker Miller Training Institute; member of the Board of Directors of Human Dignity and Humiliation Studies; and co-editor of *The Complexity of Connection*.

Elizabeth Sparks, PhD, is on the faculty of the Jean Baker Miller Training Institute; and Associate Professor of Counseling Psychology, Boston College.

This article is based on a presentation that was a part of the 2001 Summer Advanced Training Institute sponsored by the Jean Baker Miller Training Institute.

INTRODUCTION

We would like to think that most clinicians work in settings that are receptive to relational approaches to therapy, environments that explicitly or implicitly value the qualities of growth-fostering relationships, mutual empathy, mutuality, authenticity, where clients and clinicians regularly experience aspects of the five good things described by Jean Baker Miller (1986): zest, empowerment, clarity, sense of worth, and a desire for more connection. However, we know that many clinicians have had to be relational-cultural trailblazers, bringing Relational-Cultural Theory (RCT) into their practice of therapy, into their interactions with families and communities, into their interactions with colleagues and supervisors, and into their interactions with organizational systems. Unfortunately, most of these contexts rest on traditional theories of psychological development that suggest that healthy development follows from an evolving process of separation from relationships. As a result, these environments reinforce and reward practices that promote the development of a separate self, rather than practices that encourage relational development or growth through connection.

Judith Jordan (1997) observes that, "Normative socialization teaches that we are safer and stronger if we can exist without needing relationships" (p. 2). Normative socialization–in alignment with traditional models of psychological development–propagates the values of separation from relationship, competitive individualism, hyper-independence, and self-sufficiency (Jordan, 1999). RCT offers a new view of development, proposing that people grow through participation in mutually empathic, mutually empowering relationships. This view is supported by a substantive body of research that shows that engagement in supportive relationships throughout one's life enhances development and strengthens resilience (Spencer, 2000; Hartling & Ly, 2000). Nevertheless, most Relational-Cultural Practitioners live and work in environments that are rooted in the values of the dominant, separate-self paradigm, which perpetuates the view that independence and separation from relationship are the ultimate goals of development (Cushman, 1995; Putnam, 2000).

Taking a relational-cultural approach to therapy while working in settings that valorize separation challenges us to exercise professional and personal courage, the courage to pursue a vision of growth through connection, not only in our interactions with our clients, but also in our interactions with colleagues, supervisors, administrators, and other service providers. By taking a relational-cultural approach, we are committing ourselves to critically analyzing and transforming the systems of power, domination, subordination, and stratification that impede the health, growth, and development of all people.

In this article we will explore some of the obstacles and opportunities associated with being a Relational-Cultural Practitioner working in nonrelational settings. Specifically, we will (1) discuss a four-step model for strengthening our resistance and resilience, (2) examine three challenging examples of nonrelational working situations, and (3) identify ways to begin transforming nonrelational practices into opportunities for creating constructive change or growth through connection.

Of course we would like to offer Relational-Cultural Practioners a complete and comprehensive roadmap to optimal workplace resilience, if such a plan existed. We would like to be able to divulge "The Seven Highly Effective Habits of Successful Relational-Cultural Therapists." But, rather than offering simplistic solutions to complicated problems, we invite readers to view this article as the start of an ongoing conversation about the challenges, complexities, and promising potential of practicing RCT in nonrelational settings. Furthermore, to begin our discussion, we encourage readers to approach this topic by adopting the perspective of a "visionary pragmatist" (Collins, 2000). Visionary pragmatists hold the vision of what is possible while realistically addressing the obstacles that impede their efforts to create change. For our purposes, this means holding the vision of growth through connection while acknowledging and responding to the obstacles to connection, the forces that reward and reinforce disconnection and separation in our workplace settings.

A FRAMEWORK FOR BUILDING HEALTHY RESISTANCE AND RESILIENCE

In her book, *The Skin We're In*, Janie Ward (2000) describes a four-step model for fostering healthy resistance and resilience in African American adolescents confronted with the painful and pervasive realities of racism. Ward's model provides a method for developing constructive responses to the daily dilemmas and pernicious experiences associated with being a target of racism. In this article, we will adapt Ward's model as a framework for strengthening our resistance and resilience as Relational-Cultural Therapists working in nonrelational settings. Nonrelational settings are environments that privilege separate-self values, settings that discourage or suppress the conditions that facilitate the development of growth-fostering relationships, that impede mutual empathy, mutual empowerment, movement toward mutuality, and authenticity. Adapting Ward's model, we can take the following steps to strengthen our resilience as Relational-Cultural Therapists working in nonrelational settings (see Figure 1):

1. *Read it:* Clearly assess the context in which we are practicing a relational-cultural approach to therapy. This involves critically evaluating the possible risks associated with taking this approach in our specific working situations.
2. *Name it:* Name the practices that promote or impede our efforts to be effective relational practitioners.
3. *Oppose it:* Identify healthy options for opposing nonrelational practices.
4. *Replace it:* Take action to replace nonrelational practices with practices that foster constructive change, growth, or healing through connection, transforming practices that foster disconnectionand isolation.

FIGURE 1

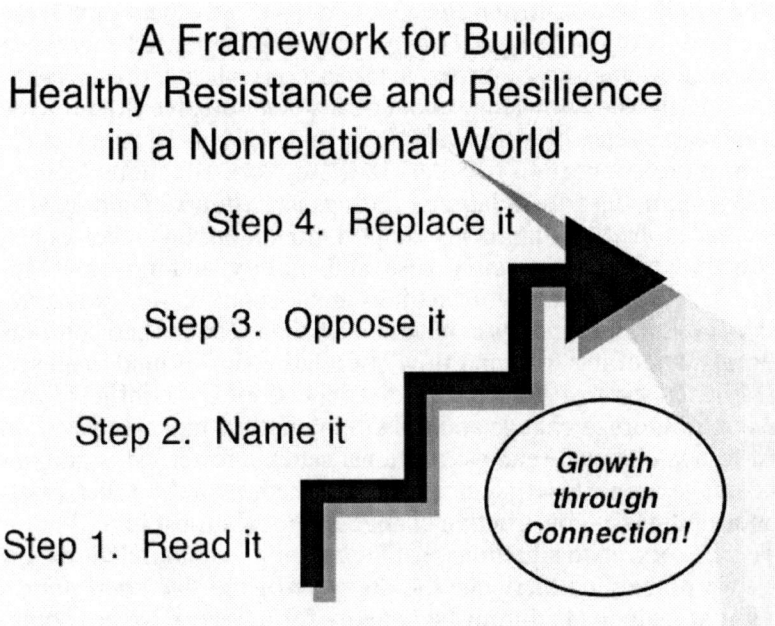

A Framework for Building Healthy Resistance and Resilience in a Nonrelational World

Step 4. Replace it
Step 3. Oppose it
Step 2. Name it
Step 1. Read it

Growth through Connection!

(Based on a model developed by Janie Ward, 2000)

Each of these steps opens a door to new possibilities for understanding and effectively addressing the challenges of working in nonrelational settings. However, it is important to note that this model was not designed to be implemented in isolation. One must have a system of support established before engaging in these steps. As always, relational practice and action work best when one connects to a group of trusted colleagues or a community of people who understand the value of relational approaches to therapy. With the help of supportive connections, we can strengthen our resilience and begin to effectively formulate ways to transform nonrelational practices utilizing these steps.

STEP 1: READING OUR WORKING SITUATIONS

How do we accurately read or assess the relational or nonrelational characteristics of our work situations? One approach is to look for the outcomes of growth-fostering relationships that should be evident in relational settings and absent in nonrelational settings. If we are working in an environment that is moving in a relational direction, an environment that values growth-fostering connection, we and others should experience aspects of the *five good things*, including increased energy for the work we are doing, empowerment to take action on behalf of our clients, increased clarity and knowledge about others and ourselves in our work setting, increased sense of worth with regard to ourselves and others, and a desire for more connection to others in these work situations (Miller, 1986). We might describe relational settings as *cultures of connection*, cultures that explicitly or implicitly support growth through relationship, mutual empowerment, responsiveness, authenticity, and movement toward mutuality. Relational work settings are not conflict free or characterized by perfect, continuous connection. Disconnections and conflicts are natural parts of the "ebb and flow" of relationships found in all settings (Miller & Stiver, 1994). In fact, disconnections and conflict are essential contributors to change and growth in relationships. However, in contrast to nonrelational settings, relational settings foster the conditions that encourage people to work through disconnections and conflict, creating opportunities for constructive change in the relationship.

If we are working in situations that are moving in a nonrelational direction, we probably experience the opposite of the *five good things*, which might include (1) diminished energy for the work we are doing, (2) feeling disempowered or stifled in our ability to take action on behalf of our clients, ourselves, or others, (3) less clarity and more confusion about others and ourselves, (4) diminished sense of worth, and (5) a desire to withdraw from or defend against relationships in these settings. We might describe nonrelational settings as *cultures of disconnection*, cultures that primarily operate on the values of the separate-self paradigm, e.g., competitive individualism, self-sufficiency, or where relational practice is devalued, discounted, or ignored. Some cultures of disconnection exhibit rigid systems of dominant-subordinate, power-over relationships sustained by covert or overt efforts to shame, blame, silence, or isolate subordinates who question the power-holders or the power structure. Other workplace cultures may provide a facade of connection, while missing essential ingredients that facilitate authentic connection and growth, such as embracing conflict for constructive change. Still other work cultures may foment an atmosphere of disconnection by inflicting excessive, relentless demands on everyone in the culture. As a result, all relational energy is cannibalized by overwhelming caseloads, inadequate resources, or constant crises.

It is important to remember that the descriptions of relational and nonrelational settings outlined in this article represent simplified generalizations of complex, multilayered, multidimensional workplace dynamics. By using the terms relational and nonrelational, we risk falling into the trap of binary thinking (Walker, 2002), inappropriately reading work settings as either relationally "good" or relationally "bad." This type of thinking will derail our efforts to create constructive change. All work situations involve complex sets of relationships and these relationships manifest a spectrum of relational strengths, weaknesses, and struggles in varying degrees at various times. Rather than classifying our work environments in binary terms, we can honor and embrace the complexities of our work situations and, as in therapy, we can focus on the *movement in relationship*, movement along a *continuum of connection* (see Figure 2). In addition, just as we can use our relational skills to read and respond to the complexities of working with a wide range of challenging clients, we can use our relational skills to read and respond to the complexities of working in a wide range of challenging environments. We can use our skills to become aware of and empathic with the strategies of survival (i.e., strategies of disconnection; Miller & Stiver, 1994) that are triggered in ourselves and others when working in difficult settings, and use these insights to begin to facilitate movement or constructive change in these work environments.

For example, a newly employed clinician at a substance abuse treatment center became aware of many practices in her clinic that routinely left her and her colleagues in varying states of disconnection and isola-

FIGURE 2

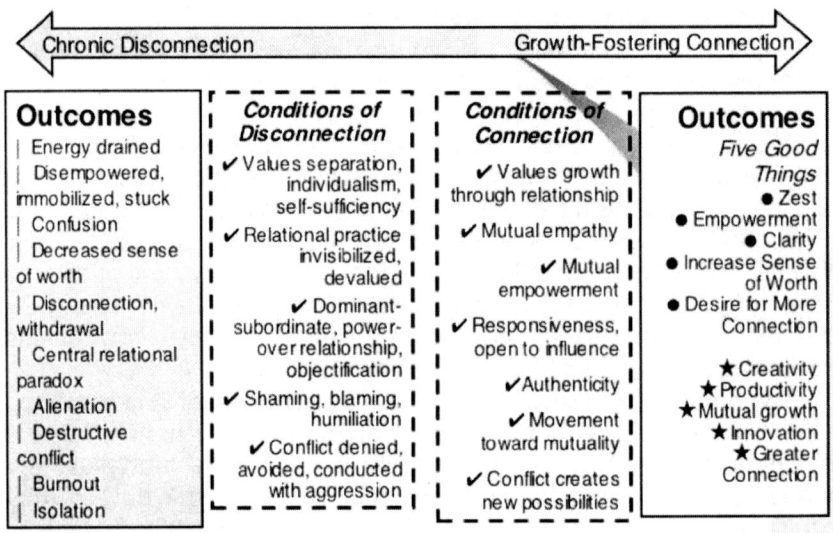

tion, including a rigidly hierarchical administration that appeared to limit collaboration, dialogue, and interaction among clinicians, supervisors, and administrators; that kept all employees under constant surveillance, and withheld information regarding difficult situations that occurred within the agency. After several months of observing these practices, this clinician learned about a devastating event that may have triggered or intensified this organization's climate of disconnection. In the year prior to the clinician's employment, the director of the agency committed suicide. The discovery of this information helped the clinician determine that a number of the nonrelational practices she observed were strategies of survival (Miller & Stiver, 1997) adopted in response to the unspeakable loss of a beloved leader, a disaster that left the surviving administrators feeling helpless, depressed, or ashamed of their inability to prevent the tragedy. This information proved essential for the clinician to empathize with nonrelational practices, in this case organizational strategies of survival, and begin to formulate resourceful and relational responses to this challenging work environment.

STEP 2:
NAME THE PRACTICES THAT PROMOTE OR IMPEDE CONNECTION

If we can clearly read the complexities of the situations in which we work, we can begin to name the practices that promote or impede our ability to be effective Relational-Cultural Practioners in various work settings. Today, many therapists work in multiple settings, or work cultures defined by numerous social, political, and professional influences. Each situation demonstrates specific configurations of relational and nonrelational practices unique to that particular setting. To explore some of the practices that occur in these work settings, we will examine three generalized types of work cultures that reflect nonrelational practices:

1. *Hierarchical cultures* that depend on rigid stratification and power-over maneuvers to manage and control individuals.
2. *Pseudo-relational cultures* that appear to value relationships, while failing to establish essential practices that promote authentic connection.
3. *Survival cultures* that are consumed by chronic crises and distress.

Again, we can note that these three classifications are over generalizations of real work situations, yet they provide a starting point to begin our discussion of the challenges and opportunities for change that can be found in these types of working environments.

HIERARCHICAL CULTURES

We are likely to encounter hierarchical cultures in academic settings, hospital settings, research institutions, and other professional organizations that have traditionally supposed that optimal workplace productivity is achieved through managing, directing, and controlling subordinates. Traditional hierarchical cultures reflect highly stratified, dominant-subordinate, one-way (i.e., nonmutual) relationships, where information and influence flow from the top down. These organizations reward and glorify individual achievement–acquired through applying power-over others–and undervalue or "invisibilize" relational practices that are essential to effectively completing the work in these settings, such as collaborative action, power-with others, open communication, relational awareness, mutual responsiveness, etc. (Fletcher, 1999). Often, dominants control subordinates by employing power-over maneuvers, such as covert or overt shaming, blaming, silencing, or isolating those who question the system or the power-holders. In particular, they manage and discourage conflict through these maneuvers. Jean Baker Miller (1976) observed, dominant-subordinate systems simultaneously suppress, deny, or avoid conflict and create the conditions that produce conflict. As a result, conflict is regularly submerged and thus perpetuated in hierarchical cultures.

Within these settings, subordinates may adopt various strategies of survival that allow them to sustain working relationships by keeping substantial parts of their experience out of relationship with those who hold power over them. RCT terms this phenomena the *central relational paradox* (Miller & Stiver, 1997). In order to keep the relationships that are available, individuals keep significant parts of their experience out of relationship. For example, a clinician may adopt the strategy of avoiding honest discussions about difficult client issues because her supervisor has used his power over her to shame or degrade her. In another setting, a scholar may sacrifice her interest in collaborative research efforts to satisfy a hierarchical academic structure that rewards individual achievement and single authorship, and devalues collaborative research.

In these cultures, clinicians must use significant energy to navigate and respond to expectations or the demands of the hierarchy and protect themselves from exposing their vulnerabilities to possible criticism or attack. The following vignette offers an example of the challenges of being a Relational-Cultural Practitioner in a hierarchical setting.

Vignette 1: A Hierarchical Culture

Paula is a staff psychologist at a private psychiatric hospital (The West Side Institute) located in a prestigious suburb near Chicago. She is a recent graduate from a well-known counseling psychology program, and this is her first job as a licensed psychologist. During her doctoral training, Paula developed expertise in a relational-cultural approach to therapy, and specialized in working with women who had histories of childhood and adult sexual abuse. She was very excited about securing the job at the West Side Institute because they had a Women's Unit that was based on the tenets of the Relational-Cultural Model. Paula was overjoyed that she would finally work in a setting that understood, valued, and practiced a relational approach.

About two years after Paula joined the staff at the Institute, a number of problematic situations occurred that caused her a great deal of distress. For the last few months, she had been having difficulty with some of the decisions that the new Medical Director, Dr. Jones, was making with regard to the management of patient care on the Women's Unit. Although Dr. Jones never articulated his feelings about the relational perspective directly to her, Paula overheard him telling a colleague that Relational-Cultural Theory was "just a lot of fluff." He seemed to strongly believe in and value the cognitive-behavioral approach to psychotherapy, and made it clear that he wanted the clinicians on the Women's Unit to strictly adhere to this theoretical perspective. Dr. Jones also didn't support the efforts being made by the Women's Unit staff to develop a milieu that would facilitate patient involvement in decision-making. He questioned many of the practices used in the milieu, and was critical of the time required for the necessary unit meetings and contact time among patients and staff that would make this sort of a milieu a reality.

The way in which power was handled within the Institute became quite clear to Paula. She knew that the medical director was responsible for all patient care within the hospital, and that he made all final decisions. Usually, Dr. Jones was willing to consult with the heads of the Psychology and Nursing Departments; however, this was strictly advisory and sometimes, he declined to take their advice.

After a particularly difficult meeting between the Women's Unit staff and the Medical Director, Paula approached the Chief Psychologist about her concerns. She expressed her frustration with Dr. Jones's attitude and decisions, which she felt undermined the atmosphere of respect and mutuality that the staff on the Women's Unit were trying to establish. Although sympathetic, the Chief Psychologist felt that it was best to simply adjust to the decisions of the Medical Director and to structure the milieu on the unit according to his expectations.

Paula has accurately read her work situation (Step 1) and is aware that she is attempting to work in a relational way within a hierarchical system that is nonrelational (Step 2). She realizes that relational practice is devalued, and that conflict is both denied and avoided. Paula must figure out a way to increase the conditions of connection in her work environment, as she facilitates small movements towards mutuality.

Opportunities for Change in Hierarchical Cultures

While there may be many opportunities for creating change in hierarchical cultures, Relational-Cultural Practioners must carefully consider the real risks associated with taking action to transform nonrelational practices in these settings (see Figure 3). In consultation with colleagues, practitioners can begin to think about relational possibilities for initiating change, which will improve the quality of the services she or he provides, benefiting clients as well as the organization as a whole. For example, creating change in a hierarchical culture may mean finding ways to make the value of relational practice more visible, such as demonstrating that effective relational practice can serve clients better–and in the end may save the organization money, time, or reduce the organization's risk of liability. Creating change may mean finding ways to make "micro" movements toward mutuality in relationships, helping the power-holders in the organization see that mutuality in relationships enhances communication within the organization preventing costly problems, improves client satisfaction, and/or increases employee job satisfaction and retention. Creating change may mean helping the power-holders in the organization see the value of creating conditions that allow all members of organization to honestly examine the challenges of the work they are doing, and foster conditions that encourage the staff to address difficulties

FIGURE 3

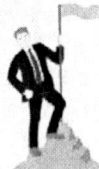

Traditional Hierarchical Culture

Challenges
- Relational practice often invisibilized, devalued.
- One-way relationships, nonmutual relationships.
- Power-over, controlling relationships; the central relational paradox.
- Conflict controlled, suppressed, denied, conducted with aggression.

Opportunities
- Change may mean making relational practice visible and valued.
- Change may mean making micro movements toward mutuality.
- Change may mean gradually creating conditions for greater authenticity: building mutual empathy, supported vulnerability.

or conflicts as opportunities for constructive change that will benefit the organization and the clients it serves. With the support of others, a Relational-Cultural Practitioner can assess the risks of taking action to transform practices in a hierarchical culture and tailor these actions to effectively create constructive movement in these settings.

Paula was concerned about taking too great a risk as she struggled to move her work environment towards greater connection and mutuality. Therefore, she chose strategies that were subtle, but which she felt would increase the visibility of the positive benefits of relational practice. Paula decided that she would work with the nursing staff on the Women's Unit to develop a Grand Rounds presentation describing how their unit facilitated patient empowerment. She also developed an evaluation project to study the effectiveness of the relational practice in reducing patient recidivism. She knew that if she could demonstrate empirically that relational practice was highly effective in reducing patients' symptomatology and increasing their ability to remain in the community (and therefore *out* of the hospital), the Medical Director and other clinical staff at the hospital would begin to appreciate the validity of this approach. After two years of implementing these strategies for change, Paula's efforts were successful. She had finally gotten Dr. Jones to accept the validity of the approach. He now realized that relational practice not only improved treatment effectiveness, but it also enhanced the hospital's reputation. This ultimately translated into financial gain, which for Dr. Jones was the bottom line.

Pseudo-Relational Cultures

Some clinicians would describe their workplace cultures as generally "nice," that is, "relational" because people in the organization appear to value having good relationships and act accordingly. However, "being nice" should not be confused with, or used as a definition of, relational practice. Being nice is about being courteous or polite. Of course relational practitioners can be nice, but relational practice is not primarily about being nice. Relational practice is about working with the complexities of relationship, which include working through differences, disconnections, and conflicts, while holding and deepening the relationship. When clinicians engage in polite behavior without addressing differences or conflicts, the outcome can be an *illusion of connection,* rather than authentic connection.

Work environments that encourage polite, courteous forms of behavior without addressing differences, disconnections, or conflicts may be creating a *pseudo-relational culture*. A pseudo-relational culture can develop in workplaces that are sincerely concerned about the quality of human relationships, such as institutions with religious affiliations, community service agencies, grassroots organizations, and volunteer groups, where individuals in the organization make it a priority to have compassion and caring in relationships with others. Unfortunately, the desire to have "nice" relationships at all times may foment an environment of superficiality, where people feel they must keep difficult aspects of their experience (e.g., disagreements, discussions of difference, conflict, etc.) out of the relationship to stay in connection. Again this situation illustrates the central relational paradox. Pseudo-relational cultures suppress, deny, or avoid differences and conflicts in order to maintain the illusion of connection. As a consequence, this type of culture can lead to the loss of authenticity, thus impairing the development of growth-fostering relationships.

Vignette #2: A Pseudo-Relational Culture

Susan, a psychologist with a background in substance abuse prevention, recently began working in a college counseling center at a small, but highly regarded coed liberal arts college in the Midwest. The college, a church-based institution, had a history of producing outstanding academic achievement within a context of caring and compassionate interpersonal relationships. However, after a few years working at the college, Susan began to suspect that relationships were maintained at the "cost" of denying and avoiding any real conflict. It was a "culture of niceness" where the staff was discouraged from expressing strong differences of opinion or disagreements.

Like many academic institutions around the country, this college was experiencing the growing consequences of high-risk drinking on campus, including vandalism, disruptive behavior, injury accidents, interpersonal violence, sexual assault, and even alcohol poisoning. However, a casual, "boys will be boys" attitude existed in response to excessive drinking, and many students took pride in having their college identified as a "party school."

In particular, Susan observed that several faculty members knew about gatherings on campus where underage students were often engaging in high-risk drinking activities. These faculty members chose not to inform the college administrators about these gatherings, even though they knew that these parties were strictly against college policy and they were aware that an increasing number of students had been treated in the infirmary for alcohol-related accidents and injuries in recent years. In addition, some faculty members altered exam schedules to allow students extra time to recover from party weekends.

When Susan asked a prominent professor about faculty attitudes regarding the growing number of student alcohol-related problems on campus, he respectfully suggested that most of the faculty felt alcohol problems were not their concern. In other words, student services held sole responsibility for dealing with alcohol problems, and any attempts to change this practice–especially expecting faculty to be more actively engaged in preventing these problems–would only create irritation among the faculty, who feel overburdened by "more important academic issues."

Susan knew that existing practices typically left the counseling center in the position of cleaning up the wreckage left in the wake of high-risk drinking so she wanted to encourage more faculty and other staff members to collaborate to prevent alcohol problems on campus. However, she also knew that attempting to change existing attitudes and practices might trigger heated disputes about student alcohol use, disputes that rarely surfaced in this "culture of niceness." Furthermore, she recognized that anyone attempting to change the status quo regarding alcohol use could quickly become discounted as a complainer, a prohibitionist, or simply a campus-wide "party-pooper."

Susan read some of the specific challenges in her work situation and began to wonder how she could begin to build bridges between faculty and other staff members that would contribute to efforts to prevent the consequences of high-risk drinking on campus.

Opportunities for Creating Change in Pseudo-Relational Cultures

A pseudo-relational culture offers many potential opportunities for transformation because these cultures value relationships and healthy interactions, at least at a surface level (see Figure 4). In fact, avoidance of interpersonal struggles or conflict in a pseudo-relational culture may be indicative of the degree to which individuals in the culture value connection *and* fear losing relationships. In these settings, change may mean recognizing that all relationships move through connections and disconnections toward growth, recognizing the natural ebb and flow of relationships (Miller & Stiver, 1994). Change may mean making micro-movements toward authenticity, finding constructive and safe ways to be real, especially with regard to disconnections or conflict. Irene Stiver suggested therapists can find something authentic to say in response to a conflict with a client that will move the relationship forward, by finding

FIGURE 4

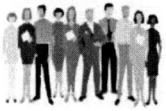 Pseudo-Relational Culture

Challenges
- Relationship "appears" to be valued, illusion of connection.
- Keeping parts of oneself out of relationship in order to keep relationships; central relational paradox.
- Conflict is viewed as a threat to relationship; conflict is suppressed, denied, avoided.

Opportunities
- Change may mean recognizing that all relationships move through connections and disconnections toward growth.
- Change may mean "micro" movements toward mutuality and authenticity; test the waters.
- Change may mean viewing conflict as a way to create the possibility of change.

"one true thing" to say. Perhaps change in pseudo-relational cultures involves regularly finding "one true thing" to say when confronted with difficult interactions with others, a true thing that moves us and our organizations toward greater authenticity in relationships. Similar to hierarchical cultures, change may also mean helping others view conflict as a way to create new possibilities for change that will enhance services for clients or increase the effectiveness of the organization. Yet, once again, we need to work in alliance with others and weigh the risks when taking action in these types of settings.

Susan began her efforts to overcome the challenges of working in pseudo-relational culture by taking many small steps. First, she began to build alliances with professionals working in similar settings who were dealing with the same concerns and problems. This approach allowed her to gain new ideas for engaging faculty members in efforts to prevent substance abuse problems. Second, she identified and began to develop relationships with influential faculty members sympathetic to the issue. These faculty members could use their influence to attract additional involvement by other faculty members. Third, Susan invited student advocates to speak to their professors about the disruptions they had experienced as a result of alcohol or drug use on campus. The students asked their professors to support or participate in changes that would reduce these problems on campus.

These small steps began the process of breaking through the pseudo-relational culture of niceness, creating constructive change. Susan was successful in organizing a task force that included faculty, staff, and students to address the problem of alcohol use on campus. After two years of hard work by the task force, she was able to document that the incidences of acute alcohol poisoning and alcohol-related assaults among the student population were significantly reduced.

Survival Cultures

In the field of mental health, *survival cultures* may represent one of the most common forms of work cultures. In survival cultures, clinicians become chronically overwhelmed or overburdened by the demands of their jobs. Consequently, they may abandon relational behaviors, viewing them as unnecessary or as poor use of time. In these conditions, clinicians become nonrelational by default because the goal of the work is to survive the immediate crisis or complete the urgent task. In an attempt to respond to excessive demands, clinicians in these settings may adopt the nonmutual practice of self-sacrifice or selfless giving in a heroic attempt to meet the needs of their clients. Ultimately, self-sacrifice does not work. Perpetual self-sacrifice eventually takes its toll on the therapist, putting her or him on the path of illness, burnout, and other forms of personal or professional disaster. Community mental health agencies, social services, child protection agencies, and other community organizations coping with enormous caseloads and limited economic support can easily become survival cultures.

Vignette #3: A Survival Culture

Agnes is a psychotherapist who has worked for five years in the Mental Health Department of a community health center (The Heights), located in a low-income neighborhood of Philadelphia, Pennsylvania. Economic, racial, and social conditions create many problems for residents and they do not have the services and amenities that help many middle- and upper-class people. The clients at the Heights are African American and Latino ethnic-minorities as well as Caucasians who live in two large public housing developments that are located near the clinic. Most of these families cope with a number of problems. The parents often have chronic medical conditions (such as diabetes, hypertension, HIV, substance abuse) and are not always fully compliant with medical follow-up. The families are generally large and at least one or more of the children have medical complications secondary to premature births: low birth weights, asthma, and/or prenatal exposure to toxic substances.

The families also experience a number of difficulties due to the environmental conditions within which they live. Violence is an everyday occurrence in the neighborhood, and a majority of the children have been either direct victims or witnesses to violent altercations on the streets. Domestic violence is also a significant problem, although many of the victims are reluctant to self-identify. Because of these family problems and environmental hazards, the mental health department staff treat many children who exhibit symptoms associated with post-traumatic stress disorder and attention deficit/hyperactivity disorder. They have behavioral, emotional, and learning problems and are typically involved with a number of different institutional systems.

Agnes has spent the last five years working with these children and their families. She has had a commitment to helping multiproblem, disenfranchised families for as long as she can remember. Agnes spent much of her graduate training learning how to provide culturally competent services to poor, ethnic-minority children, and generally feels very rewarded by her work at the Heights.

Over the last few years, Agnes' workload has gradually increased. The Heights has been facing serious financial difficulties, and the clinical director of the mental health department has experienced a lot of pressure from the executive director to balance the budget. For Agnes and the other clinicians, this has meant increasing their caseloads and cutting back on the non-billable hours (such as making collateral telephone calls or attending meetings with other providers on the cases). According to the clinical director, Agnes and her fellow clinicians have to do this collateral work in addition to keeping up with the weekly billable hour requirement.

Agnes was beginning to feel tired and drained at work. She likes her colleagues and they generally get along well. But everyone is so busy that they really never have time to sit down and talk to each other about their work. The department is supposed to have weekly staff meetings; however, many of the clinicians are too busy to attend, and even the clinical director often finds it necessary to cancel staff meetings in order to deal with other, more pressing, issues. Agnes prides herself in providing sensitive, effective psychotherapy to her clients, and she enjoys working from a feminist perspective. Nevertheless, lately, she has been feeling too tired and depleted to handle her caseload, and she just didn't know what she should do about the situation.

The mental health department at the Heights has become a *survival culture*. Agnes and her fellow clinicians are aware of the complications involved in trying to maintain relationships in their work setting, however, because of the stress involved in meeting their clients' multiple needs, there just doesn't seem to be sufficient energy left to do anything to change the situation.

Opportunities for Creating Change in Survival Cultures

Survival cultures can be transformed into environments that support the well-being and growth of clients, as well as the clinicians who serve them. In these settings, change may mean helping administrators recognize that relational practice contributes to the overall effectiveness of therapy or reduces the likelihood that clients will need long-term or intensive forms of treatment (see Figure 5). The situation will begin to change once administrators and staff understand that the benefits of moving toward mutuality in relationships, which may include increased employee job satisfaction and retention, and reduced stress, burnout, and/or employee health care costs. Change can also occur through promoting collective action and organizing individuals to challenge the social/cultural/political devaluation of relational skills, which is manifested in our society as low salaries for mental health and social service employees, inadequate funding, and unrealistic demands on service providers. Unfortunately, working in a survival culture consumes so much time that individual clinicians rarely have energy to devote to changing the system. Consequently, connection, collaboration, and collective action may be the essential keys to transforming these environments.

Many of Agnes's coworkers became fed-up with the situation, and were leaving to take jobs at other agencies. Although tired and discouraged at times, Agnes wanted to continue her work at the Heights and hoped to find a way to move her work environment toward increased connection and mutuality. Agnes knew, however, that if she was going to stay, she needed more support. So she joined a peer supervision group comprising like-minded clinicians where she could share the challenges and highlights of her work. She also wanted to become more actively involved in facilitating systemic-level change, so she joined the social action group within her professional organization that was advocating for increased funding for social services. These were small steps that Agnes took to sustain herself through this difficult period. She hoped

FIGURE 5
Survival Culture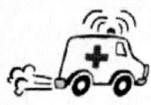

Challenges	Opportunities
λ Overwhelmed with work, nonrelational by default, chronic and pervasive nonmutuality, self-sacrificing, selfless giving.	λ Change may mean recognizing the value of relationships at all levels.
λ No structure to support relational behavior.	λ Change may mean movement toward mutuality at all levels, building mutually beneficial relationships.
λ Chronic crisis mode, burnout, focus on survival.	λ Change may mean collective action to challenge the social/cultural/political devaluation of relationships.

that in time, the systemic-level changes she was working so diligently to bring about would make a difference in the work environment, not only at the Heights, but also at other community-based agencies servicing high-risk, low-income populations.

STEP 3:
HEALTHY AND UNHEALTHY OPTIONS
FOR OPPOSITION

Whether we work in a hierarchical, pseudo-relational, or survival culture, or in some combination of these, we can begin to identify ways to oppose nonrelational practices that inhibit our being effective workers. The third step of our model involves identifying options for opposition. In particular, Janie Ward (2000) observes that there are healthy and unhealthy options for opposition. Depending on the context, unhealthy opposition results in pernicious disconnection, alienation, or isolation, resulting in harm to ourselves or others (see Figure 6). Unhealthy opposition may lead us to attack others or to become the target of attacks, such as harassment, humiliation, or other forms of persecution. Unhealthy opposition can increase our feelings of powerlessness and rage, which can trigger aggressive action in others and ourselves. Instances of workplace violence that have occurred over the last decade may be extreme examples of unhealthy opposition to nonrelational workplace practices.

Ideally, healthy opposition leads us toward constructive movement and change. It can move us in the direction of growth-fostering relationships that enhance authenticity, mutuality, mutual empathy, and mutual empowerment for ourselves, our clients, and the organization in which we work. Healthy opposition also means "waging good conflict" (Miller, 1976), conflict that is respectful and empathic with those with whom we disagree, resisting the temptation to separate ourselves by degrading, dismissing, or objectifying them as human beings. Healthy opposition involves holding the potential or vision of connection in the relationship while creating the conditions in which movement, change, or growth can occur in the situation.

Joyce Fletcher (1999), who has explored the benefits of relational practice in the workplace, offers the four following strategies that exemplify healthy options for opposition. Some of these overlap with Janie Ward's recommendations (2000):

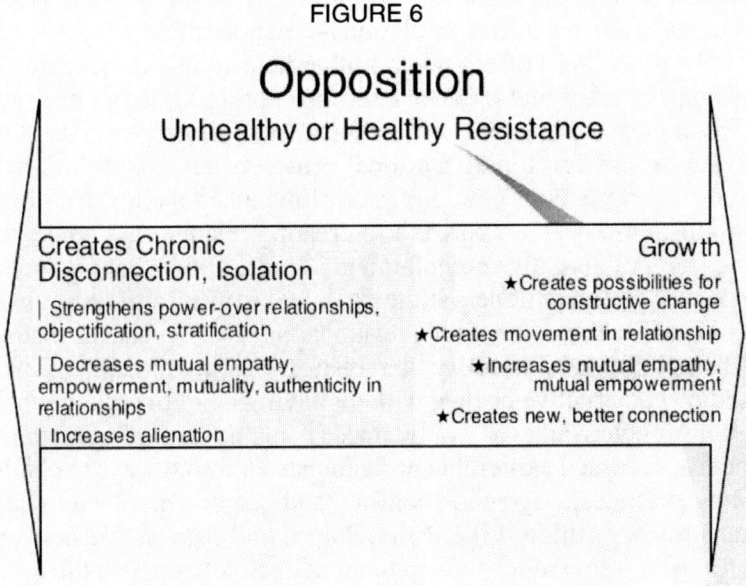

FIGURE 6

1. *Naming:* Calling attention to relational practices at work that contribute to the effectiveness of ourselves, others, and the organization.
2. *Norming:* Calling attention to the organizational norms that are not relational, norms that do not enhance the effectiveness of individuals, the services provided in the organization, or the organization.
3. *Negotiating:* Making others more aware of the value of the relational work and negotiating the conditions in which one can successfully do this work, emphasizing that relational work is *real* work and it benefits clients, the organization, and the bottom line.
4. *Networking:* Forming communities of allies to encourage and foster relational practice in the situations in which we work. As Fletcher states "Relational practitioners who have been made to feel inadequate, naive, or ashamed for their efforts to work in a context of mutuality, often find it difficult to 'know what they know'. . . A number of relational practitioners have found that forming a support group inside or outside the immediate work environment is helpful and empowering." (Fletcher, 1999; p. 130-131)

Fletcher's suggestions can help clinicians begin to formulate successful ways to transform nonrelational practices in their work settings. Judith Jordan (2002) offers several other helpful recommendations for opposing nonrelational practices and promoting systemic change, including increasing awareness of the process of disempowerment in organizations and developing a critical consciousness about internalized sources of oppression. One group of clinicians developed a critically conscious, empowered approach to creating change that could be described as "collaborative complaining." This involved having members of a network of practitioners strategically take turns initiating conversations in staff meetings about nonrelational practices, practices that inhibited their ability to be effective therapists. By taking turns, the clinicians promoted constructive change without having an individual member of the group singled out as a "troublemaker." In this example, and the three vignettes discussed earlier, the protagonists all found ways to challenge existing practices, wage good conflict, and become involved in healthy options for opposition. Like Paula, Susan, and Agnes, this network of practitioners found allies to help them collectively oppose the nonrelational, status quo practices in their work environments.

STEP 4:
A RELATIONAL APPROACH TO REPLACING NONRELATIONAL PRACTICES

The final step of our model is taking action, replacing nonrelational practices with practices that facilitate movement, constructive change, mutuality, mutual empathy, mutual empowerment, greater authenticity, or growth through connection for ourselves, our clients, and others with whom we interact in our work situations. To take action we must be sure we have done our homework and anticipated the risks and consequences of creating change. We must be sure that our relational resources are in place to provide us with support throughout the process of taking action. In addition, we must continue to sharpen and refine our relational skills, relational awareness, empathic engagement, and abilities to facilitate movement and growth in relationships. Just as these skills can be used to facilitate healing and growth in therapy, they can also help us bring about constructive change in challenging workplace settings.

While we may wish to replace the nonrelational practices in our work environments overnight, once again we must remind ourselves to be visionary pragmatists (Collins, 2000). Sometimes we can take giant leaps, but often we can be even more effective if we take *small steps,* which can ultimately lay the groundwork for larger, systemic change. Debra Meyerson and Joyce Fletcher (2000) developed the notion of "small wins" to describe the process of initiating a series of incremental changes to transform values, norms, or practices in business settings. Some people may be motivated by the image of creating small wins. Others may prefer the noncompetitive image of taking small steps to generate constructive movement in a workplace. A small steps, or small wins, approach permits us to "test the waters" to verify our assessment of the risks and impact of replacing nonrelational practices. Small steps allow us to adjust our efforts quickly whenever we need to rethink our strategies. This approach allows us to become more precise in formulating ideas for action, constructing plans that will appropriately fit the demands of the particular situation. Furthermore, small steps can create a ripple effect that extends the positive impact of our efforts beyond our immediate work environment into the larger organization and sometimes into the community.

Most importantly, we must not take these small steps alone! Relational- Cultural Practitioners need support and encouragement whenever they are working in nonrelational settings. Participating in a supportive community helps us formulate new and more effective ways to bring about change in our work settings. Participating in a supportive community strengthens our resilience in the face of daunting institutionalized practices that glorify or reward individual achievement, competitive individualism, power-over tactics, stratification, disconnection, and/or separation. In our vignettes, each protagonist took small steps designed to bring about change in her work environment. With the help of others, they gradually moved towards the goal of increasing the visibility of their relational practice, and found various ways to demonstrate its value and effectiveness to those in powerful positions who could initiate and further support the institutional change process.

CONCLUSIONS

Working as a Relational-Cultural Practitioner in nonrelational settings can be very challenging. It is often difficult to believe that change is possible within these settings, particularly in light of the often intractable way that the status quo is reinforced and maintained. In this article we have provided a framework to help you begin to think about ways of supporting relational practice within these types of nonrelational work environments. We have offered examples of possible strategies that could be used to bring about change, one small step at a time. It is important to remember that change is never accomplished without some risk, and the approach that we have described highlights the need to make a careful assessment of the risks involved in one's particular situation before determining the strategy that might be most effective. We encourage you to stay connected to a supportive network as you engage in healthy resistance, and to find like-minded colleagues who can assist you in developing increased resilience. With creativity and perseverance, positive movement towards a more relational culture is possible in most situations. But even when this is not possible, finding ways to sustain and support oneself until a different work environment can be obtained is essential. Participating in a supportive community amplifies our energy to take action to replace nonrelational practices with practices that allow us to be more effective Relational-Cultural Therapists, providing the best service to our clients, our organizations, and our communities.

REFERENCES

Collins, P. H. (2000). Black feminist thought: Knowledge, consciousness, and the politics of empowerment. New York: Routledge.

Cushman, P. (1995). Constructing the self, constructing America: A cultural history of psychotherapy. Reading, MA: Addison-Wesley.

Fletcher, J. K. (1999). Disappearing acts: Gender, power, and relational practice at work. Cambridge, MA: MIT Press.

Hartling, L. M., & Ly, J. (2000). Relational references: A selected bibliography of theory, research, and applications. Project Report, No. 7. Wellesley, MA: Stone Center Working Paper Series.

Jordan, J. V. (1997). Relational therapy in a nonrelational world. Work in Progress, No. 79. Wellesley, MA: Stone Center Working Paper Series.

Jordan, J. V. (1999). Toward connection and competence. Work in Progress, No. 83. Wellesley, MA: Stone Center Working Paper Series.

Jordan, J. V. (2002). Learning at the margin: New models of strength. Work in Progress, No. 98. Wellesley, MA: Stone Center Working Paper Series.

Meyerson, D. E., & Fletcher, J. K. (2000). A modest manifesto for shattering the glass ceiling. Harvard Business Review, 78(1), 127-136.

Miller, J. B. (1976). Toward a new psychology of women. Boston, Beacon Press.

Miller, J. B. (1986). What do we mean by relationships? Work in Progress, No. 22. Wellesley, MA: Stone Center Working Paper Series.

Miller, J. B., & Stiver, I. P. (1994). Movement in therapy: Honoring the "strategies of disconnection." Work in Progress, No. 65. Wellesley, MA: Stone Center Working Paper Series.

Miller, J. B., & Stiver, I. P. (1997). The healing connection: How women form relationships in therapy and in life. Boston: Beacon Press.

Putnam, R. D. (2000). Bowling alone: The collapse and revival of American community. New York: Simon & Schuster.

Spencer, R. (2000). A comparison of relational psychologies. Project Report, No. 5. Wellesley, MA: Stone Center Working Paper Series.

Walker, M. (2002). How does therapy heal when the culture hurts? Work in Progress, No. 95. Wellesley, MA: Stone Center Working Paper Series.

Ward, J. V. (2000). The Skin we're in: Teaching our children to be emotionally strong, socially smart, and spiritually connected. New York: Free Press.

Learning at the Margin: New Models of Strength

Judith V. Jordan

SUMMARY. This article was originally presented at the April, 2000 Learning from Women Conference sponsored by the Harvard Medical School and the Jean Baker Miller Training Institute. It explores the ways in which marginalization and the use of power-over maneuvers and privilege contribute to disconnection at a personal and societal level. Strength in vulnerability is proposed as an alternative to strength in isolation. The author suggests that courage is created in connection and the distorting effects of the myth of the separate-self must be challenged in order to appreciate the power of connection. This article examines specific ways to resist the disconnecting and disempowering effects of hyper-individualistic values both in and out of therapy.

Judith V. Jordan, PhD, is Founding Scholar and Director of the Jean Baker Miller Training Institute and Co-Director of Working Connections Project; Assistant Professor, Harvard Medical School; co-author of *Women's Growth in Connection*; editor of *Women's Growth in Diversity*; and co-editor of *The Complexity of Connection*, JBMTI.

INTRODUCTION

Understanding the dynamics of power and privilege is central to any discussion of the personal and societal effects of connection and disconnection. Awareness of one's own position in the dominant hierarchy is also an essential piece of this inquiry. I am committed to working to improve the lot of all women and men, and as a woman I experience the marginalization of gender; yet I stand squarely in the privileged center in many ways, and I have much unearned advantage in my life. Just to name some of my unearned advantage: I am white (in a white dominant, racist culture); I was born into a middle class family (education, enough money, a lot of safety in a small town); and I am metabolically and accidentally thin and tall in a world that esteems thin and tall. My list of unearned privilege is quite lengthy, but when I try to come up with unearned disadvantage I am hard put to find it. At one time being a woman felt like a source of disadvantage, but more and more this feels like unearned advantage! I have a worrying, slightly depressive chemistry, I'm over 55, aging and aching, and as an adolescent my height (6 feet tall) seemed like a terrible disadvantage; still none of these things represents a major, lasting source of marginalization or disadvantage.

A range of marginalizations exists in this world from traumatic oppression to dismissal or trivialization. Some places at the margin are places of oppression. Some are also places of powerful perspective and strength. All are potentially places of disconnection, fear, and pain. And all marginalization is an assault on our humanity and our dignity. Some people develop amazing capacities to resist and transform the dehumanizing, objectifying forces that marginalize. Some cannot.

Patricia Hill Collins (1990) notes, "each individual derives varying amounts of penalty and privilege from the multiple systems of oppression that frame everyone's lives" (p. 229). Audre Lorde (1984) observed, "the true focus of revolutionary change is not merely the oppressive situation which we seek to escape, but that piece of the oppressor which is planted deep within each of us" (p. 123). There are few pure victims or oppressors, few who exist only in the dominant, privileged mode or only at the margin. In working on the problems of objectification and dehumanization, we must recognize and "own" our places of privilege. In order to move toward empathy, true connection, and toward a model of deep human caring, we must acknowledge our vulnerability and find ways to support the vulnerability of others.

Margin and center are not actual, real places or static categories; nonetheless they are useful metaphors to address imbalances of power, privilege, and oppression (hooks, 1984).

I don't want to idealize or valorize marginalized groups. The pain and woundedness of being pushed to the margin, excluded, devalued, stigmatized, or oppressed are nothing to celebrate. Marginalization poses a major threat to our sense of connection, to our authenticity, often to our physical well-being.

In what Patrician Hill Collins (1990) calls the "matrix of domination," "people become objectified into certain categories such as race, gender, economic class, and sexual orientation. Once categorized, they are either relegated to outsider status, with the dominant society shoring up its strength, maintaining its values, and affirming its rightful place as the measuring stick by which all others are to be judged" (p. 228). Powerful social groups, including the mental health profession, name what is normal and what is deviant, what is inferior and what is superior. The power to name is profound and most of us in the helping professions must acknowledge our own positions of power in this area.

Let us look at what happens to marginalized groups, whether they are women, people of color, gays and lesbians, working class individuals, or welfare moms, and so forth. People at the margin are defined as "objects": they are seen as being at the margin because of some essential failure of character or effort. The myth of meritocracy and the myth of the level playing field support this distorted understanding of privilege. That is, people who have not "made it" deserve the place they occupy. While the notion of center and margin is not a dichotomous category, the process of marginalization suggests that if you are at the margin, you are incompetent until proven otherwise; if you are from a marginalized group and are successful in terms of the center's definition, you are the exception to the rule; if you are not successful, it proves that you *are* the problem and are inferior in some core way. In fact people at the margin are actively socialized to believe that they *have* failed, that they *are* the problem and occupy a position of disadvantage because of inherent unworthiness. This is more than a "lose-lose" situation. This is at the core of disempowerment and disconnection.

The group at the center makes the rules and names the situations and conditions of privilege and disadvantage. The prevailing attitude toward those who do not enjoy the privilege and power in a given system is one of denigration. In mental health parlance we pathologize the experience of people at the margin. This is obvious in blatant sexism, racism, or heterosexism, where broad strokes of negative stereotypes are aimed at individuals with various characteristics who are deemed inferior by the naming group.

As Joyce Fletcher (1999) notes, more subtle invalidation occurs in some of the approaches of "helping" or dealing with people at the margin. One approach is that of *assimilation*: let's bring "these people" in, fix them, help them be more like us (the dominant group). Inherent in this approach is the notion that "we" have nothing to learn; we do not need to change. A second approach is one of *accommodation*: we will accommodate to the unusual characteristics of this group. For instance, vis-à-vis women, we will accommodate to their need to spend time with children by creating a mommy track. Or we develop a welfare system that punishes and blames mothers who are working hard to raise their children. But the hidden belief is that women are weak; they need special treatment and this supportive treatment is made very visible and is resented (unlike the abundant invisible support given the dominant group). A third approach on the part of the dominant group is to *celebrate difference*: in this approach the group continues to be marginalized and treated as "different." While at first glance this can look like acknowledgment and honoring of the special qualities of the group, it is often a kind of dismissive treatment; women are "good with people," "let's put them in human resources departments or in childcare," and pay them next to nothing. Each of these models suggests change is one-directional. Those at the center, in power, dictate the norms and standards and impose them on the people with less power who need to change.

An alternative approach, consistent with the relational model of mutuality is one of *transformative* change through mutual learning (Meyerson & Fletcher, 2000). It is built on a two-way openness to change, tolerance for uncertainty, empathic listening, and a conviction that all real movement and growth promoting change must be in relationship and mutual. Furthermore, it depends on the belief that engagement with difference is enhancing to all participants. Ultimately, change depends on transformative learning for all participants through mutual empathy and empowerment between center and margin; assimilation and accommodation produce only unilateral change. We are looking for change at a systemic level. But forces operant in the current organization of the culture, that, in a shorthand way we can call the forces of patriarchy or ethics of domination, interfere with the creation of real paths of mutual change and transformation in almost all segments of the society.

People are pushed to the margin to the extent that they differ from the dominant group. Isolating, silencing, shaming, disconnecting, and stigmatizing are all used to disempower them. At the extreme, people who are different are traumatized with emotional abuse, racism, anti-Semitism, heterosexism and are often forced to disconnect from their culture of origin. Severed connections among people on the margin and between the margin and the center serve the needs for power of the dominant group. These severed connections ultimately sap the energy and vitality of the whole culture.

The existing models of strength in this culture, both in and out of the mental health field, follow from the values of the dominant, privileged group. As Jean Baker Miller (1976) noted, "In Western society men are encouraged to dread, abhor or deny feeling weak or helpless, whereas women are encouraged to cultivate this state of being" (p. 29). Yet feelings of weakness are universal; we all have them. The denial of weakness and gendered notions of strength distort both women and men. Models of strength, both in our psychological theories and in the culture at large, emphasize strength in separation, supremacy of thought over feeling, objectification, and instrumentality. In general, there is an assumption of the primacy of separation and individualism and a belief that control and power over others is the route to safety and well-being.

Alan Johnson (1997) calls it "the great lie of patriarchy." While this is supposedly a model of strength, it basically rests on a fear-based model that denies vulnerability. As bell hooks (2000) notes, "fear is the primary force upholding structures of domination. It promotes the desire for separation, the desire not to be known. When we are taught that safety lies always with sameness, then difference of any kind will appear as threat. The choice to love is a choice to connect to find ourselves in the other" (p. 93). A clinical vignette sheds light on some of this:

Brenda's father was dying of cancer. He was stoic, and financially extremely successful. When his health began to deteriorate he did not let his family know how sick he was. Brenda's mother later told her "he didn't want you to worry." Brenda noted, "Maybe he *was* trying to 'protect me,' but I think he was also caught in being a strong man to the end. And I felt abandoned. His version of being strong felt weak to me. I wish he could have let me know his vulnerability. I wanted to be there for him. And the way he set it up, he died before I even knew he was terminally ill. He was alone with his fear and now I'm alone with my sadness at not having been able to be with him."

RESISTANCE

A notion of *strength in vulnerability,* or *supported vulnerability,* is a core concept in rethinking our understanding of strength (Jordan, 1992). This notion involves openness to being moved. The first step in transforming existing models of strength is in resisting disempowering definitions of self and worth that emerge from those at the center. bell hooks (1990) notes that the margin can be "more than a state of deprivation." It is also the site of "radical openness and possibility, a site of resistance"; the chosen margin becomes a "site of transformation" (p. 22). Patricia Hill Collins (1990) noted, "empowerment involves rejecting the dimension of knowledge whether personal, cultural, or institutional that perpetuates objectification and dehumanization" (p. 230). These constitute the most horrible forms of disconnection and isolation. When we feel most separate from others and from the flow of life we are at most risk. "Oppressed people resist by identifying themselves as subjects, by defining their reality, shaping their new identity, naming their history, telling their story" (ibid., p. 229).

Resistance involves transforming disconnection into stronger connection, and creating communities of resistance. At the core of resistance lies the goal of shifting the dominant culture from a culture of "power-over" and separation to a culture of empathy, love, and mutuality (Jordan, 1997), from a culture that celebrates the elevation of the individual to a culture that emphasizes community.

Often people who enjoy more of the benefits of the center position suggest, I think quite cynically, that people at the margin can be leaders in social change because "they have less to lose." While it is true they may have more to *gain*, people who are marginalized actually put themselves at great risk when they begin to confront the injurious practices of the dominant center: they are bombed, lynched, shamed, arrested, beaten, and more. More benignly, those who protest or complain are sometimes referred to as participating in a "cult of victimization" or a "culture of complaint." I have suggested in other places that we might celebrate the art of complaining as an act of creative resistance to destructive stereotypes (Jordan, 2000). But we must know that rarely will our complaints be welcome. We will be labeled whiners, complainers, or political troublemakers, lacking humor and balance.

People at the margin have been wounded, injured, and disempowered by existing power structures but many have also developed incredible powers of survival, resistance, and ultimately transformation. How does someone on the margin retain voice, connection, impact, and visibility?

How does anyone, marginalized or not, become an agent of change? The forces of denigration are abundant. Girls are rewarded for silence and obedience. They are objectified. In the times of slavery psychiatry had a diagnosis of drapetomania, "an insane desire to run away." It was not enough to torture and kill those who sought freedom, the culture also had to pathologize the very human need for freedom itself. Today our professions often pathologize the need for connection by calling women too dependent, too needy, or too emotional. Objectifying and shaming are powerful tools to isolate and silence perceptions of reality and value systems that diverge from the mainstream.

Shame is the experience of feeling unworthy of empathic response from another; one senses that one's being is not worthy of love or connection and that one's love is also not adequate. In shame, people move into isolation and disconnection; both of these experiences contribute to silence, a loss of voice. The spiral of shame arises as we are unable to speak our authentic experience to another for fear of rejection and judgment; we move into more isolation. Ultimately, we find ourselves in what Jean Baker Miller (1998) calls "condemned isolation," the experience of feeling outside the human community, isolated, immobilized, and self-blaming. The antidote is to be respectfully and empathically "listened" back into voice and ultimately back into connection.

Shaming acts to control, silence, and disempower people, to create doubt about their constructions of reality and to elevate the dominant set of values. While outright force is used to intimidate and silence (witness the prevalence of lynching in the post-civil war south), harassment, objectification, and shaming are still rampant in attempting to disempower and frighten marginalized groups. For instance, as I was preparing this article, an article in *The Boston Globe* noted that hate crimes against gays and lesbians in Massachusetts increased by 20% in 1999. According to the Gay, Lesbian, and Straight Education Network, high school students hear anti-gay comments an average of 26 times a day. Ninety-seven percent of the time teachers who witness these comments do nothing. Gay, lesbian, bisexual, and transgendered persons represent about 30% of all documented teenage suicides (*The Boston Globe*, April 11, 2000). This is about the effects of shaming and controlling.

In another article two days later (April 13, 2000), *The Globe* reported that there is more targeting of black women by U.S. Customs officials for strip searches for drugs, this despite data documenting that this group is *less* likely than any other to bear illegal hidden drugs. Black women U.S. citizens are *nine* times as likely as white American women to undergo strip searches but less than *half* as likely to be concealing illegal drugs. What is that about if not shaming, marginalizing, and objectifying? In the face of such blatantly unjust and oppressive intrusions on personhood the individual has little recourse. But clearly communities of resistance, in this case a group of black women who decided to sue the U.S. Customs and publicize these injustices, can make a difference.

What I have learned in talking with and reading about people who *have* made a difference, who have contributed to social change from various conditions of marginalization, is that connection, love informed by a desire for justice, and community action are the most effective responses to marginalization. Resistance is a first step that paves the way for transformation.

While this is an oversimplification, I tend to think of a five-step-process of resisting disempowerment and disconnection. I might add that these steps serve not just to promote systemic change but personal change as well.

1. *Awareness:* First there must be awareness of the process of disempowerment and then the capacity to name it.
2. *Naming:* In naming it, we also try to "source" it, say where is it coming from. This helps us move out of a tendency of self-blame or accepting the blame that others cast on us, which is part of the shaming, silencing strategy of disempowerment. Coming into voice and out of the isolation of self-blame and internalized shaming brings about movement and sense of possibility.
3. *Connecting:* As a third step we connect, to find allies, to find encouragement, to create a validating, growth-fostering community. While I name this as step three, connecting actually precedes and follows from all these steps. It is essential to the process of empowerment and resistance.
4. *Critical consciousness:* This develops in the context of an encouraging community. With our allies, we can begin to strategically confront and challenge crippling stereotypes or internalized sources of oppression. This may involve using anger in the service of justice.
5. *Assess the risk in the context of connection:* Facing the challenge of disempowerment and disconnection can occur only in the context of strong enough connection. While there is never any absolute safety and we must always assess the risk involved in our efforts to confront hostile or disempowering forces, the development of strong connection stands at the core.

Janie Ward and Tracy Robinson have developed a wonderful schema to develop "resistance for liberation" for African American adolescent girls (Robinson & Ward, 1991), and Carol Gilligan (1982) and her colleagues have given us enormous insights into the development of political resistance.

When Rosa Parks, with great courage and integrity, refused to surrender her seat to a white man on a bus in Montgomery, Alabama in December, 1955, sparking a major chapter in the civil rights movement, she was not alone, but was already a part of a larger movement for social justice, a movement that both empowered her and gained courage from her courage. It is partly the American way to make the communal, relational forces that support the courage of individuals invisible. We prefer to perpetuate the image of isolated heroes that reinforces the status quo of hyper-individualism. Appreciating the relational roots of courage in no way undercuts the absolute courage of the individual but it strengthens our sense that change occurs within social contexts, not within the lonely but brave hearts of separate people (Jordan, 1990).

The idea that strength occurs in connection, not separation, is a powerful challenge to the dominant paradigm. Disconnection from ourselves and from others is one of the potential risks and costs of marginalization. Creation of internalized self-hatred, shame, lack of self-worth, and trauma is in large part what marginalization is about.

NEW MODELS OF STRENGTH

As Jean Baker Miller noted in 1976, "women's great desire for affiliation is both a fundamental strength, essential for social advance and at the same time the inevitable source of many of women's current problems" (p. 99). Some have said that resistance and revolution begin with the self, in the self. I would say they begin with a redefinition of the self, a movement toward apprehending that relationship, not separation, is primary in people's lives and toward claiming the strength found in connection not in separation. This profound shift moves away from believing that separation is the primary human condition to perceiving growth-fostering relationships as the core source of safety and meaning in people's lives.

I would like to suggest that our new models of strength emphasize the qualities of courage, care (love and empathy), compassion, community, good conflict, and competence (The Six Cs). Courage, which I have written about previously (Jordan, 1990), involves the capacity to act meaningfully and with integrity in the face of acknowledged vulnerability and fear. The root word, *cor*, means heart–coming from the heart. Courage is not a trait encapsulated in the solitary individual. It is constantly created in connection through encouragement. We see this in the stories of change agents time and time again. This creation of courage is one of the most important things we can do for one another.

As Tessa Thompson, a teen victim of date violence who now helps other victims said, "The courage to give is the fuel to live" (Waldman, 2000, p. 78). Most importantly, we encourage one another to be able to move into conflict, to stand in a place of difference, to create what bell hooks (1990) calls "an oppositional world view" (p. 15). We need to "listen one another into voice" and into courage. As Brenda Ueland notes, "critical listeners dry you up" (Ueland, 1999). In moving out of objectification and isolation, toward mutual respect and growth, we help each other *see clearly, speak strongly, and seek allies*.

STRENGTH IN VULNERABILITY

Human vulnerability is a fact of life. Because we love, we inevitably suffer loss. Furthermore, we all live in aging bodies, we are subject to physical illnesses and psychological injury, we die, we control far less of our lives than our control-driven culture would have us believe. Psychological vulnerability, or openness and responsiveness, is essential to authentic connection and mutuality. It is the place of our growing edge. Strength in vulnerability may seem like a paradox, but with a sense of supported vulnerability, when others see, know, and respect our vulnerability, we are open to real growth (Jordan, 1992). If we find collective support we gain the courage to stay open and responsive rather than resorting to the use of power over others or encapsulation and disconnection.

When connections fail us, we often seek protection through "power-over" rather than "power-with" actions. There are times when discernment allows individuals to decide when "protective inauthenticity" may be called for. Clearly we all make decisions on a moment-to-moment basis about what to share, disclose, or what access to allow. Authenticity is not a moral imperative to "be totally honest." Authenticity is a complex process of assessing one's own risk and gauging the impact of certain truths on the other while respecting the needs of the relationship.

Joyce Fletcher (1999) talks about making relational practice visible and of taking small risks in hierarchical systems. This involves challenging systems in which relational practice and competence is made invisible, taken for granted, or marginalized. When people feel unsafe we become less authentic and this often spirals into increasing disconnection and isolation. Maureen Walker has said, "Marginality is about social disconnection, personal and political violation, and pain. It can be and often is disabling. It can be and often is a place of piercing perspicacity; as bell hooks has suggested, a position from which to discern, confront, and subvert the machinations and the delusions of the center. It is often on the margins that we encounter and experience the transformational gifts that enliven and strengthen our relational capacity" (Walker, personal communication).

THERAPY

I believe that a key to these transformational gifts is in the supported vulnerability that develops in some of these places on the margin. I do not want to glorify places of suffering. Maureen Walker recently told me of an article called "Why I Want to Bite R. D. Laing." It was about Laing's tendency to idealize emotional suffering. The relational model recognizes our need to move from an illusory sense of self-sufficiency and a tendency to deny vulnerability toward realization of supported vulnerability. In the central movement of mutual empathy in therapy, both therapist and client are open to being affected and moved. Using the relational model, therapists are invited to be more real, more vulnerable, more mutual. This is not about factual self-disclosure, equality, or losing the larger frame of the therapeutic relationship, but about being deeply and respectfully engaged in a process of change. In opening to being moved emotionally, the therapist ideally practices strength in vulnerability.

Traditional models prescribe a kind of distance, mystification, or opaqueness (and please do not believe these models are a thing of the past; they are alive and well and influencing many therapists). Therapists practicing with new models move out of the "certainty" of old ways of doing therapy. New models invite us to move toward our own personal edge, to our professional edge. This shift does not mean moving out of a zone of safety for both client and therapist; feeling "safe enough" is essential to building healing connection, and protection of our clients is core to our ethical principles. But, it means moving out of a kind of false certainty into more open learning with our clients, which can lead us to a difficult sense of vulnerability and possible shame.

Expectations for therapists can be especially shaming when we are starting out in the field, when our vulnerability is often extreme. I still remember my very first therapy hour with my very first client. My entire intern class sat behind a one-way mirror taping the session so that we could go over it together in minute detail later with a brilliant but incredibly critical supervisor. I remember being so nervous I could barely talk (my mouth was stone dry) and I remember looking at the video later, thinking, if you didn't know I was the therapist, you would surely think the client was the therapist and I the client. I said the right things like "How can I can help you?" (I probably should have asked, "How can I *possibly* help you?"). I was a wreck. The client did a great job helping me be (and appear) more competent than I was. That also reminded me of another time when a new client, in her shame about coming into therapy, said to me "If you really knew me you wouldn't want to work with me in therapy." At that time the thought crossed my mind, "If you really knew *me* you wouldn't want to be in therapy with *me*!"

As therapists we need to move out of images of ourselves as perfectly empathic. The creation and protection of inflated self-images often becomes the source of profound isolation. We have to face our own limitations. We cannot assume that the client is the only one who connects in less than perfect ways. Often movement out of connection for therapists occurs around experiences of uncertainty or vulnerability. These are often the occasions when our expectations for ourselves, our expectations to be able to *do* something helpful, leave us feeling helpless or flawed. Often we hold unrealistic images of what a "good" therapist should be.

I must constantly avail myself of the wisdom of valued colleagues. I remember one consultation early in my work with the relational model. This consultation occurred when I was experiencing a particularly rough time with a client and I was in a particularly vulnerable period in my life. I was trying so hard to be "strong" for her. And I remember Irene Stiver doing a consultation; Irene often comments on the phenomenon of how well our clients know us and how well they protect us from what they know. I remember Irene saying, "Judy she knows you're going through something rough. She doesn't need to know the details but she needs confirmation from you that you are a little preoccupied, a little disconnected." Of course she did, and as soon as I was able to do that our impasse softened. I had this image of being strong, consistent, rising above my own human limits and I shut down and disconnected when I couldn't match this image.

Shame sometimes keeps us from seeking the dialogue or consultation that could help us stay in connection with our clients during these hard times. The dominant, white middle-class culture's overvaluation of control and certainty carries over into the culture of therapy. As therapists, we often become armored or defensive and disconnected when we are uncertain, ashamed, and anxious. As therapists, we need to ask ourselves what our places of fear and unworthiness are? What happens when clients seek to meet us psychologically where we feel most vulnerable?

Certain clients will take us to our growing edge more than others. I remember one young woman who actually left treatment before I thought we were finished. We worked together for several years. She had been in a fair amount of therapy before she began seeing me; most of these therapies lasted about six months and then some impasse would develop. She kept in touch with one former therapist whom she valued and trusted. In the early months of our work together, she engaged in self-destructive cutting and ingesting pills. I was worried, felt vulnerable, and sometimes helpless and not sure if I could help her.

Although I did not know it at the time, she confided to this former therapist that I was the first person she trusted enough to share her chaos with. The therapist commented to her, "So I guess Judy should feel complimented that you're winding up hacking yourself to pieces because you trust her so much!" She just kept taking me to my edge and hers, too; she would talk about needing to walk the edge and needing not to be alone. When I reached the limit of what I could tolerate and felt her safety was at stake, I let her know I could go no further. I stated this in terms of my limitations. Sometimes I'd say, "I know you need to go there to feel connected and alive but I just can't handle how frightened I get when you're that vulnerable and I worry about your safety. Can we try to figure something else out that is respectful of both of our needs and will also protect this relationship?"

Years after she stopped therapy with me and had gone on to do some extraordinary work with another younger therapist, she contacted me; I thought to probably rake me over the coals. She actually called to say that she knew I'd had a really hard time with the vulnerability of working with her but that seeing that I cared, that my caring made me feel scared sometimes, was really helpful to her. She commented that my willingness to *not* go on "automatic pilot" as other therapists had done (in her words "covering their own asses") and my willingness to be vulnerable with her meant I had some trust in her, in our relationship and in our ability to work through some of the places of fear.

Therapists sometimes are kept from communicating what they're actually doing in therapy (even when they're doing very fine work) because they fear censure and shaming from colleagues. In talking about my therapeutic work with many groups of clinicians over the years, many people say, "Oh yes, of course, this is the way I've always done it but I've always been in the closet with it or I can't tell other people what I'm doing because they'll think I'm doing it wrong or there's something wrong with me." They often add, "But my heart won't let me do it the way I was taught, with all the distance, objectivity, and non-responsiveness." Shame isolates us professionally and keeps us from growing in connection.

I might add that as teachers and supervisors in the field of mental health we are also vulnerable to shame. Recently, I gave a two-day workshop in Pennsylvania and as part of it I did a small segment on sexuality about which I felt a little nervous, vulnerable, and exposed. I thought it went okay but I was glad when that segment was over. As I glanced at the evaluations at the end of the day, most were pretty positive but one comment jumped out at me: "Great conference except for that inane diatribe on sexuality!"

My recurring question, professionally and personally, is "What facilitates healthy change and growth in people's lives?" This exploration of the margin and vulnerability is yet another variant of that question. If we are in touch with our vulnerability, it seems to me we can move either into fear and shame or into humility and connection. I believe humility and compassion are essential to real connection, to real healing, and to change in both the therapist and the client. And the movement to humility depends on being in an empathic context. We need to accept our limits, not as major faults and places of shame, but as part of accepting who we are as human beings. We need to practice self-empathy and empathy for others. People tend to strive for specialness or they become encapsulated in egocentricity or narcissism when connections fail. Isolation breeds striving for superiority or "power over." When we have to assume a position of "better than," we move out of mutual connection. This need to feel "better than," or lack of belief in connection, in part creates the need for power-over others.

Therapists too must work from a place of caring and humility. This is, after all, humble work. We have few, if any, absolute answers; we bring caring, we practice fluid expertise with our clients, a back and forth of learning and growing; we invoke certain relational skills and qualities of attention and awareness; we bring commitment to the well-being of the client. Our own lives sometimes do not reflect the best of our own understanding and hopes; and sometimes that is a source of shame. For instance, I am painfully aware of how tenaciously I cling to the privilege of the center in many ways despite my very deep and real appreciation of the people who can choose the margin as a place of protest, justice, and integrity.

In a recent workshop on shame, a group of therapists and mothers wrote anonymously about their experiences of shame. Many therapists spoke about the shame of being seen as less than perfect, sometimes simply as too human, by clients. I was reminded of Harry Stack Sullivan's observation that "everyone is much more simply human than otherwise" (Sullivan, 1953, p. 32). One woman wrote about being in a loud tug-of-war with her three-year-old over a bag of Oreos in the supermarket, both of them literally on their hands and knees pulling as hard and stubbornly as they could when a client of hers walked down the aisle.

For therapists who are making use of new models of therapy, who are, in some ways, at the margin, the processes that are invaluable for any group at the margin also apply: Connect, find encouragement, develop critical consciousness toward disempowering belief systems, work on your shame, become part of something bigger, join a group to explore alternative ways of working, make a commitment to the healing relationship, and make a commitment to understand your work with trusted colleagues and allies. You do not have to be a relational expert; I can't even begin to tell you what a nonexpert I am in relationships (my colleagues here could, however!) and yet my commitment to understanding and expanding our ability to connect is deep.

VIGNETTES

I want to close by sharing several vignettes of women who in different ways came from the margin and acted with encouragement for the empowerment of others. They represent strength in vulnerability and they represent to me the power of service, spirit, and love.

Kris Rondeau

Kris Rondeau (material from personal communication and Hoerr, 1997) who played a prominent part in the 1988 victory of the Harvard Union of Clerical and Technical Workers, described herself as a small town hick from a working-class family who was very depressed as an adolescent. She also described herself as committed to correcting social injustice. After graduating from college, Kris got a job as a lab assistant at Harvard Medical School where some fragmented movement toward unionization was already occurring; Kris was interested. What Kris objected to most at Harvard was the coldness of the institution. She wanted to help construct a union that helped people, made them feel they were a part of something important.

She felt that anger was a poor organizing tool. Instead, she and her colleague-friends wanted to "teach people to have confidence in themselves, to take responsibility for changing their situation in life, to form a community so strong that nobody on the outside would chip away individual self-confidence and frighten members into submission" (Hoerr, 1997, p. 86).

The anti-union campaign that Harvard mounted was built on creating fear and lack of self-confidence. It was big and powerful. However, the women organizers at Harvard were very persistent; Kris's husband described her as "relentless." They were also playful. For instance, when asked at a social event what she did for a living, Kris said, "I shovel shit at Harvard Medical School." To which someone responded, "Oh, that must be *good* shit."

Kris believed that the women workers wanted to be part of something more intimate, more human than Harvard management was willing to provide. The entire union organizing effort was built on connecting women with other women, on developing personal relationships with each worker. After 11 years, two lost elections, and endless denigrations from both management and traditional unions, the Harvard Union of Clerical and Technical Workers–3,500 strong, mostly women–won the election. Despite her incredible personal courage and perseverance, Kris later admitted that during much of the process, "We thought the guys were right." Her message was not to defeat or humiliate, but to transform an unjust system that would benefit both worker and institution and to do it by establishing connections.

Ella Baker

Ella Baker was one of the original organizers of the Southern Christian Leadership Conference and a driving force in the formation of SNCC (Student Nonviolent Coordinating Committee). She believed in the concept of "group-centered leadership rather than leadership-centered groups" (Grant, 1988, p. 6). She noted of Martin Luther King: ". . . the movement made the man . . . it wasn't the man who made the movement" (Grant, 1988, p. 103). Basing all of her work on "developing the strength in others," she was instrumental in drafting the SNCC statement of purpose which said: "Through nonviolence, courage displaces fear, love transforms hate, acceptance dissipates prejudice, hope ends despair, peace dominates war; faith reconciles doubt. Mutual regard cancels enmity. Love is the central motif of nonviolence" (Grant, 1988, p. 130). That about says it all!

She commented on the paradox of struggling to become part of society, the quest to belong, alongside the inevitable question about whether one really wanted "in." She asked "is this the kind of society that permits people to grow and develop according to their capacity, that gives them a sense of value, not only for themselves, but a sense of value for others?" (Grant, 1988, p. 215). Ella Baker also noted, "Struggling myself don't mean a whole lot. I've come to realize that teaching others to stand up and fight is one way my struggle survives" (Grant, 1988, p. 216).

VIGNETTE 3

A client, in speaking about her mother's dying, recently pointed out that the sick and dying are often marginalized in this culture. The Stone Center Theory group on chronic illness and disability taught me a lot about this experience (Halen, Reid-Cunningham, Snyder-Grant, Stein, & Tyson, 1999). But in reflecting on my client's comment, I began to realize a lot of this topic for me is about my mother. She taught me a lot about courage, about margins and about being thoughtful about what we do with privilege. She also taught me a great deal about vulnerability, illness, and dying. My mother was a bright, independent physician at a time when women doctors were anomalies. She devoted her whole life to various struggles to empower women. She was a birth control pioneer with Margaret Sanger, studied and wrote about syphilis, opened a free birth control clinic, and was outspoken about women's rights. She provided free care to many of the inhabitants of the rural county where we lived in Pennsylvania. She sponsored the opening of the first child guidance clinic in our area, helped find funding for young women who wanted to become doctors, and was an early proponent of socialized medicine (which did not lead to her popularity with other physicians). Many in the town were appalled by her ideas and I remember as a child occasional bomb threats, and visits from clergy who predicted (in front of me) that she would burn in hell for her ideas.

I'm sure I idealized her courage. But the one thing I remember that she feared was old age and senility. She was a fiercely independent woman and the thought of dependency on her children or others troubled her immensely. Playfully, but with a real underlying seriousness, she made a pact with her sister that if she ever became senile her sister should shoot her. And as fate would have it, this proud, fierce woman was diagnosed at 70 with Alzheimers Disease, and her sister did *not* shoot her. While her mind didn't work, her heart had an undaunting resilience. Often when someone would walk into the room after an absence of five to ten minutes, her face would light up and she would say, "Oh I'm so glad to see you. Thank you for coming." She was a connector. Then she would resume picking at her bedspread or talking to an imagined baby that was often with her.

Many people stopped coming to visit. To them she was "gone." Her downhill course lasted ten years. Two weeks before she died, her brain failed to send the command to swallow and she literally was unable to take in food and water. But her body wouldn't let go as she slipped into a coma. At midnight the night before she died, I, her youngest child and her "baby" to the end, slipped into her room and sitting with her, my hand cradling her neck in some instinctive posture of support, whispered, "I'm going to be okay... your baby's going to be okay ... we'll still be connected." At seven o' clock the next morning she quietly slipped out of life.

I don't want to glorify her illness. It was ugly, humiliating, and painful. It took a terrible toll on her and on her caregivers, although it also gave some of us a chance to show deep love. It was not a relational picnic and the long slide into the final phase of the illness was one of heart-rending fear. Ironically, in this disease that so decimates the brain and destroys so much of what we think of as the self in our culture, her heart, her connectedness and loving spirit, her relational being endured to the end, giving, teaching those who could stand to listen and bear witness.

As Maureen Walker noted (personal communication), "When we learn from models of strength on the margin, we learn something about the gifts of vulnerability." Thank you, Kris Rondeau. Thank you, Ella Baker. Thank you, Mother.

REFERENCES

Avyazian, A., & Tatum, B. (1994). Women, race and racism: A dialogue in black and white. *Work in Progress, No. 68.* Wellesley, MA: Stone Center Working Paper Series.

Belenky, M., Bond, L., & Weinstock, J. (1997). *A tradition that has no name: Nurturing the development of people, families and communities.* New York: Basic Books.

Brown, L. (1998). *Raising their voices: The politics of girls' anger.* Cambridge, MA: Harvard University Press.

Coll, C., Surrey, J., & Weingarten, K. (Eds.). (1997). *Mothering against the odds: Diverse voices of contemporary mothers.* New York: Guilford.

Collins, P. H. (1990). *Black feminist thought, knowledge, consciousness and the politics of empowerment*. Boston: Unwin Hyman.

Eldrdge, N., Mencher, J., & Slater, S. (1993). The conundrum of mutuality in psychotherapy: A lesbian dialogue. *Work in Progress, No. 62*. Wellesley, MA: Stone Center Working Paper Series.

Faderman, L. (1999). *To believe in women: What lesbians have done for America–a history*. Boston: Houghton Mifflin.

Fletcher, J. (1999). *Disappearing acts: Gender, power and relational practice at work*. Boston, MA: MIT Press.

Funiciello, T. (1993). *Tyrannay of kindness: Dismantling the welfare system to end poverty in America*. New York: Atlantic Monthly Press.

Giddings, P. (1984). *When and where I enter: The impact of black women on race and sex in America*. New York: William Morrow.

Gilligan, C. (1982). *In a different voice*. Cambridge, MA: Harvard University Press.

Grant, J. (1998). *Ella Baker: Freedom bound*. New York: John Wiley.

Halen, B., Reid-Cunningham, M., Snyder-Grant, D., Stein, K. I., & Tyson, E. (1999). Women with chronic illness: Overcoming disconnection. *Work in Progress, No. 80*. Wellesley, MA: Stone Center Working Paper Series.

Hartling, L., Rosen, W., Walker, M., & Jordan, J. (2000). Shame and humiliation: From isolation to relational transformation. *Work in Progress, No. 88*. Wellesley, MA: Stone Center Working Paper Series.

Hoerr, J. (1997). *We can't eat prestige: The women who organized Harvard*. Temple University Press: Philadelphia.

hooks, b. (2000). *All about love*. New York: William Morrow.

hooks, b. (1984). *Feminist theory: From margin to center*. Boston, MA: South End Press.

hooks, b. (1989). *Talking back: Thinking feminist, thinking black*. Boston, MA: South End Press.

hooks, b. (1990). *Yearning: Race, gender and cultural politics*. Boston, MA: South End Press.

Johnson, A. (1997). *The gender knot: Unravelling the patriarchal legacy*. Philadelphia: Temple University Press.

Jordan, J. (1989). Relational development: Therapeutic implications for empathy and shame. *Work in Progress, No. 39*. Wellesley, MA: Stone Center Working Paper Series.

Jordan, J. (1990). Courage in connection: Conflict, compassion, and creativity. *Work in Progress, No. 45*. Wellesley, MA: Stone Center Working Paper Series.

Jordan, J. (1992). Relational resilience. *Work in Progress, No. 57*. Wellesley, MA: Stone Center Working Paper Series.

Jordan, J. (Ed.). (1997). *Women's growth in diversity*. New York: Guilford.

Jordan, J. (1999). Toward connection and competence. *Work in Progress, No. 83*. Wellesley, MA: Stone Center Working Paper Series.

Jordan, J., Kaplan, A., Miller, J. B., Stiver, I., & Surrey, J. (1991). *Women's growth in connection*. New York: Guilford.

Lorde, A. (1984). *Sister outsider.* Freedom, CA: Crossing Press.
Meyerson, D., & Fletcher, J. (2000). A modest manifesto for shattering the glass ceiling. *Harvard Business Review, Jan-Feb,* 127-136.
Miller, J. B. (1976). *Toward a new psychology of women.* Beacon Press: Boston.
Miller, J. B. (1988). Connections, disconnections, and violations. *Work in Progress, No. 33.* Wellesley, MA: Working Paper Series.
Miller, J. B., & Stiver, I. (1997). *The healing connection.* Boston: Beacon Press.
Robinson, T., & Ward, J. (1991). A belief in self far greater than anyone's disbelief: Cultivating resistance among african american female adolescents. In C. Gilligan, A. Rogers, & D. Tolman (Eds.). *Women, girls, and psychotherapy: Reframing resistance* (pp. 87-103). New York: Harring Park Press.
Sullivan, H. (1953). *The interpersonal theory of psychiatry.* New York: W.W. Norton.
Tatum, B. (1997). *Why are all the black kids sitting together in the cafeteria? And other conversations about racial identity.* New York: Basic Books.
Ueland, B. (1999). Empathic listening. *Utna Reader.* December.
Waldman, J. (2000). *Teens with the courage to live.* Berkeley, CA: Conair Press.
Walker, M. (1999). Race, self, and society: Relational challenges in a culture of disconnection. *Work in Progress, No. 85.* Wellesley, MA: Stone Center Working Paper Series.

Valuing Vulnerability: New Definitions of Courage

Judith V. Jordan

SUMMARY. In a dominant, Western culture that celebrates strength in separation and holds unrealistic expectations for independent, autonomous functioning, vulnerability is seen as a handicap. This system creates the illusion of an invulnerable and separate self, and uses individualistic standards to measure a person's worth. Since these unrealistic expectations cannot be humanly attained, these controlling images become the source of shame and disconnection. RCT suggests that there is value in embracing vulnerability and in providing support, both at an individual and a societal level, for the inevitable vulnerability of all people. Rather than espousing the individual, mostly mythical, traits of a "lone hero," RCT moves us toward new and important pathways to resilience and courage through connection. A version of this article was originally presented at the 2002 *Learning from Women Conference*, co-sponsored by Harvard Medical School and the Jean Baker Miller Training Institute.

Judith V. Jordan, PhD, is Founding Scholar and Director of the Jean Baker Miller Training Institute and Co-Director of Working Connections Project; Assistant Professor, Harvard Medical School; co-author of *Women's Growth in Connection*; editor of *Women's Growth in Diversity*; and co-editor of *The Complexity of Connection*, JBMTI.

INTRODUCTION

It is always exciting to be here at the *Learning from Women Conference*, but as many of you know, this particular conference still fills me with the strangest mixture of excitement and anxiety. This year's conference seemed especially hard to prepare for. My topic, working with vulnerability and courage in connection, arose partly in response to the events of September 11th. But it seemed like these ideas have been speaking to me for a while, though unfortunately, rather softly and unclearly.

In a recent dream, I was sitting with Irene Stiver, saying that I just couldn't do this conference without her. We were sitting on a balcony of some stately looking building with a lot of people. It turned out that we were already at the conference and Irene was saying, "I'm here, I'm here." I was feeling better as she spoke to me; it was a dream image of courage in connection, if you will. Many of you may know that Irene was here for the Harvard women's conference in 2000. That day is very much with me today as it was her last professional presentation. She was diagnosed with lung cancer a week after that conference and died four months later. I want to dedicate this talk to her. I also want to dedicate it to Jean Baker Miller, another dear friend and colleague who has taught me much about courage in connection. Jean first signed me on to present at an Orthopsychiatry conference in Toronto. When I protested that I was phobic about speaking in public and asked if someone else could give the paper I wrote, Jean gently suggested we should take the notion of voice seriously. She encouraged and supported me to come into my voice.

At that conference, my short paper on empathy and the mother-daughter relationship, given with much trepidation, engendered the following question from a man in the audience: "Dr. Jordan, would you care to comment on the implications of empathy for Marxist and Capitalist systems of government?" My mouth dropped open and I started to dissociate. Then I looked at Irene on one side of me and Jan Surrey on the other for the support that I knew would be there. With their silent encouragement, I managed to say, "That's an interesting question, I'm sure you have some thoughts about that," and indeed he did. He went on to give a short talk. The man's question was profound, but I just wasn't "present" enough to grasp its significance. The Relational-Cultural Model, while very relevant to the practice of therapy and personal relationships, is not just a sweet theory about "cozy" or "nice" connection. It presents a challenge to the dominant paradigms of separation, radical individualism, certainty and images of invulnerability both in and out of therapy.

To Irene, Jean, and all of my colleagues here, I thank you for helping create the courage to try to forge new models of human development and human connection and new ways of understanding women. And to all of you, I thank you for helping to listen us into voice, for encouraging us. I share my sense of vulnerability and my hope for the power of curiosity, openness, learning, and growing in connection. This work is partly about ideas, but it is also about our hearts, our lives, our hopes, and our passions.

COURAGE IN CONNECTION

Courage is ordinarily depicted as a characteristic of the lone, separate person who defies vulnerability and fear. In a paper written in 1990, I suggested that courage, unlike macho defiance of fear, is the capacity to act meaningfully and with integrity in the face of acknowledged vulnerability. There is no real courage where vulnerability and fear are denied. According to the Oxford English Dictionary (1971), the word courage derives from the Latin root "cor" meaning, "heart" and it lists the first definition as, "the heart as the seat of feeling, thought." Traditional Eurocentric culture extols courage as a trait to be found in the solitary individual, an internal characteristic existing within a person who often faces her or his fate alone. This propagates a myth of "separate courage" rather than "courage in connection."

Seeing courage only as an internal, solitary trait eliminates an understanding of the way people help to engender and support one another's courage. It obscures the fact that we all need encouragement throughout life in order to stay vital and confident, to bring our most deep and real energy into connection. Courage involves bringing our truth into relationship. It often involves the courage to move into conflict. Bringing ourselves authentically into relationship leads to inevitable conflict around difference, and the courage to move into conflict is essential for growth and change. Courage also involves building resistance to the radical individualism of the dominant culture, challenging the definitions that are imposed on the less powerful by the more powerful, and importantly, challenging the messages that make the less powerful "the problem."

Carol Gilligan (Gilligan, Rogers, & Tolman, 1991) alerted us to the importance of political resistance in psychological theory. Janie Ward (2000) has written about the special quality of resistance for liberation for African American adolescent girls. Patricia Hill Collins (2000) notes that "the authority to define societal values is a major instrument of power." She also notes that, in resistance, "There is a refusal to accept the applied definitions and identities from the dominant group" (p. 69). In resistance, we say to the dominant culture, "you cannot define who I am or convince me that I do not belong" (ibid., p. 39).

As women and as people concerned with helping others, we need to resist the myth of the lone individual conquering nature, being master of his fate, in control, certain of and moving to a position of power over others as confirmation of his strength, and trying to maintain images of being invulnerable and independent. We need to offer models of courage that emphasize our ongoing need for connection and encouragement. Similarly, we need to challenge the construction that suggests desire for connection and need of others is the territory of weak and emotionally immature women. We need to challenge the dominant images of "power over" others, as they shape experiences of gender, race, class, and sexual orientation. We need to question the power of binary thinking that objectifies and creates opposition around difference (weak or strong, poor or rich, gay or straight, black or white).

When we have the courage to move beyond certainty and invulnerability we enter the world of learning, curiosity, and, dare I say, love. We risk the hope of becoming part of something larger, transcending the illusion of the separate self. We can enjoy the spaciousness of real humility or we can become paralyzed with shame, a sense of personal inadequacy. The need for certainty can lead to imposition of simplistic categorizations, whether they be diagnoses or social categories, which distort the experience of both the namer and the named. To be present in life and in the therapeutic relationship, we must dwell in uncertainty. In order to do this, we must tolerate our own and the other person's vulnerability and we must create safe contexts and systems in which this can happen. In individualistic systems, understanding, courage, agency, and activity are seen as existing within the individual. The failure to meet the prevailing standards of strength and goodness are seen as problems of the individual.

"Be a man" is the highest exhortation in our culture. It carries a notion of courage, strength, and pride. How often have I heard as a compliment, "You think like a man," or as a child, "You run like a boy"? A mother at a recent conference on gender came up to me at the end of one of my presentations. First, she told me that she was a longtime feminist and had tried to raise her son to think outside the usual gender boxes. She reported the following anecdote: her eight-year-old son was playing on a soccer team that had one girl who was a very skilled and competent soccer player. A player from the other team came up to this woman's son and said, "You're on a girls' team, you're a girl–you're all girls," followed by, "Neh, neh, neh," the universal taunt sound. This woman watched her son's reaction. He looked pained (the taunt had found its target) and angry, but he paused and retorted, "We are *not* girls!! We're *not* girls!" Then he paused again and the look on his face changed completely. "We're *not* girls. We're–WOMEN!!!" This boy had somehow learned resistance and perhaps the fine art of Aikido: take the energy coming at you and go with it for your own empowerment. Apparently, the bully was completely nonplussed by this response and withdrew.

VULNERABILITY

Vulnerability is defined in the Oxford English Dictionary (1971) as "susceptible of receiving wounds or physical injury; open to attack." It carries the notion of not being adequately protected, unsafe. But of course, protection is a contextual term. In certain circumstances being open and psychologically visible is essential; in other situations, armor and protection are necessary. Depending on the context in which we feel vulnerable, we may in fact be in danger and open to injury. The experience of vulnerability depends very much on the relational context. In a system of radical individualism and cutthroat competition, vulnerability is often a fear-filled experience. In a violating, non-mutual and power-over system, vulnerability is a dangerous experience. And in a stratified and oppressive society, those at the bottom are continually forced into places of vulnerability and then reminded of their vulnerability, partly as a means to intimidate and control them.

Much of the struggle associated with creating new models of development arises from language. How can we use the language of the dominant discourse, a language riddled with assumptions of separation and power over others. How can we develop new language or reframe old concepts in a context of connection? As Patricia Hill Collins (2000) said, "We are developing an epistemology of connection versus an epistemology of separation" (p. 71). In this vein, I would like to suggest that we reframe vulnerability as an experience in which we are open to the influence of others at the same time that we are open to our need for others. We feel we can bring ourselves more and more fully into relationship. There is an openness to mutual impact, a sense of being safe enough to move toward connection with others. When we are vulnerable, we are capable of being "moved" by internal affective experience, as well as being affected by other people. In an empathic or compassionate milieu, we honor emotional openness and reward trust with care and respect. Sarah Lightfoot (1999) said, "Making oneself vulnerable is an act of trust and respect, as is receiving and honoring the vulnerability of another" (p. 93). But we might also look at different kinds of vulnerability since the way we experience vulnerability is so dependent on the context within which it occurs.

Supported vulnerability occurs in relationships where one is provided the kind of caring that allows one to explore one's full range of being in a safe and mutual context (like therapy). Mutual vulnerability occurs in growth-fostering relationships where both people experience a deep connection and openness to change. Forced vulnerability involves the exercise of power over others, sometimes including humiliation, being rendered vulnerable against one's will. This is never "safe enough" vulnerability and is often experienced as traumatic vulnerability; there is too much loss of control, too much exposure, and abuse of the power differential. Humiliating others, reducing them to a state of frightened and demeaned vulnerability unfortunately plays a part in much of the subtle violence we see at personal and social levels.

ILLUSION OF INVULNERABILITY

Vulnerability, per se, is not the problem for the culture or individuals. In fact, vulnerability is an inevitable part of being alive. It is *disowned* vulnerability that creates disconnections. An openness to being affected is essential to connection; without it, people relate inauthentically, adopting roles and coming from distanced and protected places. The dominant group (white, middle-class, masculinist, straight) celebrates the illusion of invulnerability, safety in power over others, armored separation and hyper-individualism. Living in the shadow of our national trauma of 9/11, I noticed shared sadness and fear in the people I spoke with. I also noticed the anger, the knee-jerk revenge, the "How could they do this to US?" expressed more at a national and public level, rather than at an individual level. There was some sense of humiliation and counter-humiliation. It was not just the sense of pain or being in touch with the suffering that we were experiencing, it was a sense of entitlement to the illusion of invulnerability. In my therapy practice there were enormous differences in responding. One client, terrorized as a child by an older brother, could not stop crying, but she made no connection between her own early awful vulnerability and the events of

September 11th. Another woman, an abuse survivor, felt her whole life was unraveling and after four years of sobriety began drinking again. Yet another intensified her participation in *Amnesty International*. Another could not pick up the phone to call her family in New York from whom she was estranged. Several times in hearing a low-flying plane overhead both my client and I winced. We were, therapist and client, in a shared state of trauma, fear, numbness, and secondary traumatization. The veil of safety, seemingly so real but invisible (until it was threatened) for white middle-class people was suddenly ripped asunder.

The illusion of safety had never been there for citizens of Third World countries, for the mothers of inner city adolescents, for people of color, for gays and lesbians, for the mothers of the disappeared, in short, for all those who are marginalized and objectified. It was one of those invisible privileges, like male privilege or white privilege, which Peggy McIntosh (1988) addresses: *the privilege of assumed safety or invulnerability*. At the collective dominant culture level, we were all faced with the sense of our own vulnerability. Invulnerability was no longer an option. False reassurances were useless, shared terror was barely tolerable. Being present with, bearing the uncertainty and fear, acknowledging our universal vulnerability in the face of death, showing that we were touched, moved, and saddened seemed to help a little. Every client I saw had the same response: "I just wanted to be with those I loved. I felt I just wanted to touch and hug and be with my family, my friends."

The consistency of this response and some of the gender differences in the retaliation response reminded me of the classic studies of fight or flight in the face of stress. For years the dominant and only *truth* in psychology was that in the face of stress, the organism either fights or takes flight (or freezes). It has been one of the bedrock pieces of knowledge in Western psychology, the famous "fight or flight" phenomenon. It is very relevant to the issue of vulnerability. Stress involves feeling vulnerable, open to being influenced usually in aversive ways. Shelly Taylor and a group of graduate students (2000) at the University of California began to question this "universal truth" and found that the hundreds of studies of the fight or flight response to stress were done on males–male albino rats, male monkeys, and male humans. The conclusions from these studies were that in the face of stress, we either fight (are strong and courageous "real men") or we flee (are vulnerable and cowardly). Furthermore, we respond alone, based on internal traits–either lone heroes or lone wimps. When Taylor repeated these same studies on females, a very different picture emerged. In the face of stress, females tend to move toward others, to take care of, to be in close proximity, to groom and communicate. They named this the "tend and befriend" response. Taylor and associates suggest that part of this may be biologically determined, that there is a release of oxytocin for females when they are stressed or too vulnerable. Oxytocin is the hormone that is released pre- and post-birth in mothers and in all women during times of stress. While I have no doubt that biology plays a part in this, I would be hesitant, as were these authors, to explain all the gender differences in that way.

I would like to point out, which these researchers did not, that the response to stress they found does not appear to be about just "getting support" or "calling a friend to complain" (nothing wrong with either of these), but there is a "befriend" piece. In our language, it is about something mutual–reaching out to give, reaching out to receive. It is about building connection, and to stretch it a bit, I think it is about the practice of building courage in connection. This helps us cope, helps us stay in our vulnerability, helps us feel we are part of something larger than our own particular fear. It's interesting how much developmental models emphasize "growing bigger." Even in this model, we talk about growth as if it's about getting bigger or more expanded. I actually think of development as movement toward more integration, more responsiveness, more flexibility, more connection, and becoming a part of something larger. It is not the individual getting bigger, and certainly not the individual ego getting bigger. I heard two women in a line at the grocery store recently talking about mothering. They appeared to be strangers. One was a relatively new mother and the other was expecting her first child. The new mother was glowing and talking to the slightly anxious expectant mother and she said, "Being a mother is the most powerful thing I have ever done. You feel so small compared to your child and it's so wonderful. You're not the center."

DOMINANT IMAGES OF CONTROL

The prescriptions for white, middle-class, heterosexual males are: be in control, be certain, be agentic, be a fighter, be at the center, and don't be vulnerable, too emotional or needy. The good news is that only 20% of the population is now made up of this group; the bad news is they still hold most of the power. In these role prescriptions, there is an illusion of separation, invulnerability, and certainty. I sometimes refer to four myths that serve as the underpinnings for maintaining the societal status quo in the United States, particularly:

- The myth that we are separate: "You're born alone and die alone" (any woman who has given birth might question this saying).
- The myth of a just world, or the myth of meritocracy: "We get what we deserve in life." Therefore, CEOs deserve eight million dollars a year (but welfare mothers do not deserve "handouts").
- The myth that we are invulnerable and in control: if we practice good self-care and vigilance, we will flourish.
- The myth that competition brings out the best in us and leads to the greatest productivity.

These myths support a developmental pathway of radical individualism, autonomy, self-sufficiency, and excellence achieved through competition.

To acknowledge a need for connection is to acknowledge vulnerability. We may move into narcissism and power over others when connections fail us or when the vulnerability of wanting connection is too threatening. In power-imbalanced, non-mutual, or unsafe relationships, vulnerability can become a place of fear and disconnection. The strategies of disconnection that Irene Stiver and Jean Baker Miller wrote about are developed to protect an individual's vulnerability in unsafe conditions (Miller & Stiver, 1997). Part of the work of therapy is to create conditions of connection and safety that allow people to begin to relinquish strategies of disconnection and to come back into the vulnerability that is necessary to establish authentic connection. For some, especially those who have experienced trauma, this is a very slow, small-step process. People learn through the careful attention paid to their pain, misunderstandings, and disconnections that a place of vulnerability need not always be a place of terror; it can become a place of growth, connection, and joy. Ordinary courage, the courage to move from old relational images that suggest negative consequences, to an experience of vulnerability, not knowing, and uncertainty, occur in the context of a relationship characterized by mutual empathy.

I am reminded of some therapeutic work on which I have been consulting. Karen is an inspiring, kind, and intelligent therapist with whom I always learn. The last time we talked, Karen told me of her work with a fourteen-year-old girl who is dying of a brain tumor. Karen works with the mother and daughter together. I'll call the daughter "Diane." Diane is at the end of her life and the doctors have told her that there is nothing more they can do. She is hoping she can stay alive for her fifteenth birthday because she loves birthdays. She is troubled because her friends seem to be pulling away from her. They don't know how to handle her illness, her ultimate vulnerability. She knows this but it leaves her feeling scared and lonely. Her therapist, Karen, and I talk about the possibility of convening a meeting of her friends, to help them, possibly to help them be with Diane. In the shadow of death, we therapists sometimes find a way to step out of our own well-worn paths of neutrality or our individualistic mindset of working with the patient and her internal world. Karen, the therapist, tells me she has given both mother and daughter an identical bangle bracelet for each to wear so that when they can't be physically with each other they will have the bracelet to be physically reminded of each other's love. Karen comments that she, the mother, and the daughter burst into tears when these bracelets were given. I also cry as I hear this. There is a moment of silence, of connection, of unbearable pain. I feel privileged to be part of this work of healing and love. I am reminded of this therapist's own experience of grief in losing her beloved brother to a brain tumor when he was 30. This information is not explicitly in the room with Karen and the mother and the daughter, but it is with Karen as she sits with this courageous pair. It is with me as I talk with Karen, who also exhibits tremendous courage in her work. In the meantime, the divorced father is seeking one more expert opinion. He, too, is living his love. Every parent I have ever known has talked about the loss of a child as the worst possible thing that could happen; even nonparents know that deep in their hearts. The vulnerability of being a parent is exquisite. It takes enormous courage to be open to the love and possible loss.

MUTUAL EMPATHY

Therapy is a deeply personal, alive, moving relationship of healing and change in which the connection between therapist and client serves as both the incentive and the vehicle for change (Jordan, 2001). Mutual empathy is at the core of change, and responsiveness on the part of the therapist lies at the heart of mutual empathy. This movement of caring, empathy, and deepening understanding of one's experience of the other and the relationship is nurtured in an environment of profound respect and openness to uncertainty. June Jordan (1981) once commented, "While self-respect is essential, respect for others is the key" (p. 144). The practice of mutual empathy is predicated on mutual vulnerability.

Our work suggests that isolation is the primary source of suffering and that people come into therapy with both a yearning for connection and often a terror of the vulnerability that is necessary to move into growth-fostering connection. That is, in order for empathy to lead to growth and change, the client must be able to see and feel that he/she has an impact on the therapist and their relationship, i.e., she must be empathic with the therapist being empathic with her. In this corrective relational experience she sees that she matters, that she can be effective, and that she can evoke a response. Self-empathy and empathy toward others is fostered in this movement.

Careful, considered clinical judgment guides the responsiveness of the therapist. But in this real engagement between client and therapist, where both are open to change, and are vulnerable in differing ways, there is new learning and real healing of chronic disconnection. If a disconnection occurs (and they occur all the time) and the person is heard, responded to, and made to feel that her feelings and experience matter to the other person, then the connection is strengthened and transformed. It is in the healing of these acute disconnections that we gain a sense of trustworthy connection and being effective in relationships. We rework old relational images and strategies of disconnection.

If in the past another person, often someone with more power, had not been responsive to the representation of our feelings, we learned that we cannot have an impact on the other person or the relationship, and we develop strategies of disconnection to protect our vulnerability and our real feelings. Strategies of disconnection are, in fact, strategies of safety or survival. In order to keep unacceptable, unwelcome, and vulnerable aspects of ourselves from being exposed to an uncaring, possibly violating other, we begin to disconnect from our internal experience and we begin to disconnect from authentic connection with this rejecting or hurtful other.

The vulnerability necessary to move from strategies of disconnection (protection, survival) back into the original yearning for connection is often terrifying. In fact, entry into therapy in and of itself can lead to an escalation of a person's use of strategies of disconnection. The therapist's task then is not simply to deconstruct the strategies of disconnection and push the client back toward connection. As Miller and Stiver (1997) point out, the therapist must be empathic with both the need for disconnection, the strategies of disconnection, and with the deep and ongoing yearning for connection. The therapist must honor the client's vulnerability. In addition to the personal sources of disconnection, societal sources, such as discrimination and power imbalances based on race, ethnicity, sexual orientation, and class, create enormous pain for people and must be acknowledged in the therapeutic work.

To the extent that therapy positions itself as a "power-over," "expert knows best," inaccessible, neutral, emotionally disengaged enterprise, it aligns with the dominant cultural patterns that often create chronic disconnection in the first place, at both an individual and societal level. To the extent that the therapist is open to influence from the client, is responsive, engaged and not opaque, the therapist offers resistance to the traditional therapeutic norms of separation and disconnection, and offers a kind of vulnerability to change that allows the client to see, know, and feel that she has had an impact, that she makes a difference, and that she matters. This allows the client to move back toward connection, as well as to begin to grow in places where strategies of disconnection have kept the person walled off with the illusion of invulnerability. For therapists this involves a shift in values and understanding, from a model of purely intrapsychic growth of the client, culminating in autonomous functioning, to one that provides support for the client's inevitable vulnerability and helps create the courage to connect. But responsibly resisting dominant patterns of practice and creating new therapeutic paradigms creates vulnerability for the therapist and requires a surrounding community of resistance and encouragement.

Places of mutual vulnerability are often the places of potentially great growth or impasse in therapy. For instance, when clients let us know that we have hurt them, if we stay open, we can feel empathy with that pain and feel sorry for having caused it. We can feel the vulnerability of the other person in letting us know this and we can feel our own vulnerability in having created the pain. While we often feel an easy, open empathy when the client has been hurt by someone else, when we are the source of the pain, in addition to our concern for them, we may feel shame, inadequacy, defensiveness, a pulling away, disconnecting, shutting down, or armoring. We do not want to know the pain we create for others. In our defensiveness and shame, we may abandon our clients. Staying in our own sense of vulnerability, imperfection, and remaining with the person, rather than withdrawing to maintain an image of ourselves as the "all good" therapist, leads to powerful therapeutic movement.

THERAPEUTIC AUTHENTICITY

The question of authenticity and being real in therapy is a complicated one. I have called this the question of: *"How to be real and how real to be?"* Relational authenticity is one of the building blocks of Relational-Cultural Therapy. I think schematically of the model as being like a triangle with relational authenticity, mutual empathy, and mutual empowerment/encouragement at each apex. This triad creates growth-fostering relationship characterized by the five good things (Miller, 1986). It is in our struggles with how to be real and how real to be that our own vulnerability as therapists often surfaces. But as Irene Stiver (Jordan, 1992a) noted, "I can't imagine a therapist being responsive in a growth-fostering way to the client's vulnerability without opening up our own vulnerability. We are reframing the traditional therapy style by saying that one has to be open to one's vulnerability in order to be able to foster the process. The acknowledgment of vulnerability alone is an enormous mutual experience in therapy" (p. 12). Working to be engaged and relationally authentic is about being responsive to the client, using anticipatory empathy to help us judge how, when, and to what degree our authenticity will serve the growth of the client.

Relational authenticity is not total honesty, spontaneous and complete sharing, or knee-jerk reactivity. It is not even really self-disclosure in the sense of telling one's life story or sharing personal information, although there may be some disclosure of life facts in the service of healing chronic disconnections. It is about letting clients see their real impact on us, which is a process that, again, involves enormous clinical judgment and attunement. In order to shift patterns of chronic disconnection and the negative relational images that support them, we must begin to see what impact we have on others, that we are not alone and helpless, that we can influence others, and that our feelings matter to others.

Our model suggests that chronic disconnection is the source of major pain and suffering in people's lives and the therapeutic task is to begin to help the client move back into connection with her inner experience and with others. Chronic disconnections result from the kinds of disconnections that do not allow people to have an impact, to feel they are relationally competent. In order to shift this pattern and the relational images that support it, we must begin to see what impact we have on others, that we are not alone and helpless, that we can influence others, and that our feelings matter to others. Being real on the part of both therapist and client involves a certain sense of risk or vulnerability. The client may wonder, "Will I be heard, responded to, respected?" In therapy the client develops the courage to bring herself more fully into relationship and into creative action.

THE QUESTION OF BOUNDARIES

Respect, clarity, and responsibility on the part of the therapist for the well-being of the client are essential in working with vulnerability and capture for me the values that are often tagged with the concept of "boundaries." Some of the traditional boundary concepts partake of the dominant paradigm of a separate-self, resisting influence, demarcating spheres of influence or control, in order to establish power over others as a way to ensure personal safety. It is important to remember that the "self" is a metaphor (Cushman, 1995; Jordan, 1992b). There is no such thing as a self. The bounded, separate self is a metaphor built on a model of separation rather than connection. I believe safety and psychological growth arise in good connection, not in the experience of self-sufficiency, autonomy, and boundedness. Growth-enhancing relationships depend on responsiveness, clarity, the capacity to represent one's needs and feelings, respect, and the expectation of mutuality. In helping rework old protective strategies of disconnection and relational images that support isolation, it is essential that the therapist pay attention to the safety of the client.

The shift from a separate-self paradigm to a relational-cultural paradigm makes the current boundary concept problematic. I would like to propose that we rethink the traditional concepts of boundaries, to create a model that emphasizes the following:

- clarity;
- responsiveness, not reactivity;
- safety for both participants, which importantly involves respecting a person's vulnerability and not using one's power to take advantage of another's vulnerability; mutuality (one person is not making use of the other); and
- the need for both people to stay connected with themselves, aware of their own limits and stating those limits, as well as being clear about the possible consequences if there is not respect for those limits.

There is attention to mutuality and an awareness and respect for one's own and the other person's limits. It is important to *state our limits* rather than *set limits* on others. This is about respect, responsibility, and authenticity. In stating our limits and encouraging the other to state her limits, we are providing relational information. Perhaps if we think of a boundary as a place of meeting, rather than as an armored dividing line protecting against an impinging outside world, this concept would make more sense (Jordan, 1996, 1999; Miller et al., 1999).

A CLINICAL VIGNETTE

To illustrate some of these points in working with vulnerability, I'd like to share some clinical material. Ellen is a therapist who was trained in a more traditional psychodynamic model, with some emphasis on ego psychology and object-relations theory. Recently she became interested in the Relational-Cultural Model and began to introduce aspects of it into her work. However, her ongoing peer supervision group was largely made up of more traditional psychodynamic practitioners. Ellen was struggling with how "to do therapeutic authenticity" and how to be real in therapy. She is a caring and responsible therapist who has many years of experience. She came to me for consultation because she was feeling burnt out and increasingly resentful in her practice. She then reported to me several cases in which she felt she was being responsive, mutual, and real. But what she also reported was a narrowing of her own space, a sense that she was giving more than was comfortable, disclosing too much, and feeling "devoured" by her clients. Furthermore, her peer supervision group was questioning much of what she was doing, and kept reminding her, "remember your boundaries."

She had taken the call to mutuality and authenticity as a call to engage in total open and honest reacting. As a result, she was feeling incredibly vulnerable, as if her life had to be an open book, that saying no or exploring the client's historical life material would always be hurtful and shaming. Over time she found herself disclosing more than was comfortable, wondering whose interests were being served, and feeling terribly anxious and shame-filled. The response in her supervision group made her feel even more filled with shame and she guessed following these supervisions she probably "closed down" with her clients, retreated to a more traditional stance, and disconnected.

As we talked she became aware that she was likely disconnecting even in the act of "giving" because the giving felt so imbalanced and forced. Her clients had begun to feel like her inquisitors. I wondered to myself how that must feel to her clients as well. She was caught between two values: wanting to be real, present, and vulnerable enough to grow, but not wanting to feel so exposed or ashamed. More clarification of how hard it was to integrate some of the new model with some of her original training was helpful, and we explored in some depth the importance of working with our limits, what relational authenticity means, and what kind of responsiveness best serves our clients.

Also, I shared with her some of my own learning while trying to navigate the growing edge around vulnerability–how I struggled to feel useful and protected enough for me to stay connected with myself and my client. I talked with her about my work with Cindy, someone about whom I had spoken before, but with a slightly different awareness regarding vulnerability. Cindy was a young woman who I saw many years ago. She was a courageous, creative, and challenging young woman, and one of my best and most energetic teachers. What she challenged in me was my image of myself as a certain kind of therapist and my need for certainty.

Cindy had been sexually abused by her stepfather from the ages of eight to twelve. Her efforts to alert her mother of her predicament at the time of the abuse were to no avail. In seven previous treatments she had been unable to talk about the abuse. She was labeled as suffering from paranoid schizophrenia, borderline personality disorder, and major depression. I was treating Cindy at a time (about twenty-five years ago) when I had had no training in working with trauma. Cindy had "fired" (or had been "fired" by) five previous therapists, and came to me because she had heard I was "different." She wasn't able to articulate how I was thought to be different, but she thought it had something to do with the fact that I listened better than some of her other therapists.

Shortly after starting our work together, she began to seriously question whether I really was a good listener. She found me unclear, unimaginative, and too passive, and furthermore, I really "missed the point" a lot of the time. I was–devastated might be too strong a word, but it's in that direction–by her assessment of me. She also began to call all of her former therapists to complain about me. Each time I said something stupid or "off," she would call someone to carefully describe my failure.

These other therapists, many former supervisors of mine at the hospital in which I was working, often approached me in the cafeteria to report that Cindy had called to tell them something unempathic or "stupid" that I had said in her therapy session. They would typically say, "Judy, *you* wouldn't have said *that*" and I would have to admit that I had (she was a precise recorder of my errors) and I'd get embarrassed, feel exposed, and way too vulnerable. My image of myself as a good therapist, or at least as a good listener, was being severely challenged. I would leave the cafeteria, feeling raw, anxious, and incompetent. I dealt with my vulnerability at that time by not going to the cafeteria.

Although I am not proud of this, I would often try to interpret Cindy's calls as hostility towards me, but I think the honest, bottom-line gist of most of my responses, gentle and well-intentioned though they may have been, was to somehow get her to stop exposing me. I didn't like feeling so vulnerable or so inept. Slowly I figured out that this was not really about hostility or aggression (old model thinking), but more about connection and vulnerability. This young woman had been sexually abused behind closed doors by an older authority figure, her stepfather; someone she was told was trustworthy. She had been unable to protect herself. She had been plunged into terror, shame, condemned isolation, and intolerable, traumatic vulnerability.

In this therapy relationship she was triggered. In many ways the therapy situation itself is triggering for abuse survivors. There is an invitation into vulnerability, behind closed doors, with someone who has more authority and power, and who is supposed to be trustworthy. Strategies of disconnection are naturally and inevitably heightened when entering such a situation. It is protective and appropriate for abuse survivors to feel suspicious, guarded, and anxious upon entering these situations.

Cindy, in fact, having felt safe enough to disclose the abuse, began to feel increasingly vulnerable and unsafe. Rather than bolting from the treatment, as she had done before, or moving into major traumatic disconnections, which she did occasionally, she figured out a rather creative way to make it safe enough to stay in treatment with me. She made our relationship public and she particularly illuminated all the hurts and failures for all the world to see. These hurts and failures, for her, were warning signs of impending danger and perpetration. The signals to her brain were calling out for emergency response. Despite her impulse to flee, she was able to channel that panic into creating a web of protection around her and us, composed of the other therapists she had invited indirectly into our therapy sessions. Further, she was able to alert me to the fact that she would not tolerate violation, and she also was able to bring both of us into some tolerable sense of mutual vulnerability.

A large part of my work, aside from merely staying with her in the not knowing, in the uncertainty, was also bearing my sense of shame and vulnerability. I really was trying to learn and appreciate the meaning of what some might call these enactments. I knew they were happening for good reason and it was my job, as best as I could, to figure out with her what it was all about. I think my willingness to go there with her was very important.

Before this whole dance ended, another one of my clients who worked on a suicide hotline arrived one day looking particularly smug.

She said, "Another one of your clients called the hotline last night, and when I found out you were her therapist, I couldn't contain my curiosity, so I asked her what she thought of you. She said she thought you were "smart but not very warm." She paused and said, "That's funny, I always thought you were warm but not very smart." (Ouch!)

Cindy's management of her own vulnerability and terrifying relational images left me feeling pushed out of my own comfortable, relational images of being a good empathic therapist into images of being angry, stupid, incompetent, and uncaring. But I think she had to go there partly because her own traumatic vulnerability was so great and raw and unsafe, and partly because I was not able to bring myself into more vulnerability–the vulnerability of not knowing. I kept trying to be the expert, in part because I thought it would be genuinely helpful to her, but also because I couldn't tolerate my own vulnerability, not being certain how to help her. In some ways the connection was failing her; both her relational images and my relational images were not working to bring about connection. In desperation, she moved into a kind of end-run, a kind of exercise of power when she could not find the responsiveness she needed from me.

Slowly, I better understood the wisdom of her strategy to stay connected enough, which paradoxically felt like a strategy of disconnection, and of course it was both. And as I could work with, and somewhat relinquish my need to know and my need to be, or appear to be, certain or competent, she also could begin to move into more vulnerability. Her way of helping us both stay in enough connection to begin to work was ultimately brilliant. She made her own traumatic vulnerability more tolerable by bringing our relationship into the public. As each of our strategies for survival failed, but as we were also finding some safety with each other, we slowly began to take small risks and get comfortable with our vulnerabilities. But this place of interlocking vulnerabilities and efforts to avoid them initially led to impasse. I would say this is one of the greatest places of impasse in all therapies, particularly when we are working with early chronic disconnection.

Cindy found a way to take me to one of my growing edges, away from my need to be the expert, certain, and in charge. Eventually, I found a way to be in vulnerability that did not abandon either her or my own sense of responsibility and accountability as a therapist. We began to open up to an appreciation of the connection and our impact on each other, rather than getting caught in endless control battles. As I felt defensive and anxious, I subtly but surely moved into more "power-over" maneuvers. She helped me move into more vulnerability, where she could see her impact on me. We moved from being stuck, she in her traumatic vulnerability and I in my role as expert, to learning and growing together.

Things began to shift as each of our strategies failed and we slowly, through our misfiring efforts to get to connection began to move into the complexity of our fears and hopes. But this place of interlocking vulnerabilities and our effort to avoid the vulnerability first led to impasse. The dance captured so much of the complexity of working with vulnerability. There were movements toward power tactics on both sides in an effort to avoid vulnerability, which also meant moving into disconnection. Both of us had to begin to let go of some of our strategies of survival, to take small risks, and to be open to finding out that we could forge connection where disconnection threatened. For my part, I had to really listen and let her teach me. I had to bear my own, what felt like, enforced vulnerability. I had to find a way to stay in empathy when I was being told I was hurting her. At such times, therapists can so easily move into power-over our clients, often through subtle expert maneuvers like diagnosis, distancing, constructing the problem as being all in the client, and so forth. This is a complex response, not either/or.

I had to struggle with my need to be and look effective and caring–partially to the external audience that had been created and partially to an internal audience of former supervisors who were also booing, hissing, and only very occasionally appreciative. I had to be in my own uncertainty. She evoked feelings in me that were not easy, and I in her.

Cindy had to be open enough to take the risks; she had to entertain some uncertainty in her fixed belief systems and the relational images that informed her that vulnerability leads only to being taken advantage of or violated by powerful others. We couldn't just alter that fixed, deep-in-her-bones conviction with talk; we had to live the solution, small failures followed by attuned responsiveness, to stay safe enough. She had to take in that she had an impact on me that although I was capable of getting caught in my own needs to feel competent or look good, that even though I was slow and reactive, I was trying to be responsive to her. I was not going to use some cookbook, DSM III distancing, "power-over," or artificially reassuring strategy to reassert control.

We both had to let go of our prevailing strategies of disconnection and develop more effective and nuanced ways of establishing safety in connection. We had to move out of the rigidity and stereotypy that fear engenders, and we had to appreciate our own and the other's complex needs and feelings. As the therapist, I had the responsibility to focus energy on helping Cindy to get clear. I had to help establish enough safety so that connection could happen.

In this therapeutic context, the relational images, which were predicated on an expectation of violation in response to vulnerability, could begin to shift in the direction of differentiating safe and unsafe interactions. My misattunements could come to be experienced as simple misattunements or disconnections. When reworked in the context of responsiveness and concern, they could lead to stronger connection rather than to the previous isolation of chronic disconnection and the feeling of relational helplessness. Part of Cindy's work was learning to differentiate the unsafe spaces within a safe-enough relationship, telling the difference between generally mutual and nonmutual relationships–no longer returning to the earlier relational images of global danger. Step-by-small step, we managed to do this work together. This is the work of mutual empathy and building relational resilience and relational competence.

Another client once told me, when I responded that it was very painful for me to watch her self-destructive and dangerous behavior, that I needed to "go to the edge" with her, that therapy would not work if I was standing on completely safe ground and only she was at the edge. But we had to negotiate this, and I had to state the limits of what I could tolerate. If I went too far to the edge (beyond my personal or professional safety zone), I actually couldn't stay present with her; I would be too filled with fear, resentment, or shame, unable to focus.

SHAME

Cindy and I were often derailed by shame. Shame particularly arises around vulnerability in a culture that so denies the importance and the inevitability of vulnerability. Cultures differ greatly on how they handle vulnerability (Jordan, 1989). While our North American dominant culture devalues and denigrates vulnerability, it is also invested in making sure that there is a group of vulnerable people, people who do not hold power and are prevented from gaining power. In such a situation when vulnerability arises, people often feel shame; it is a sign of weakness, unworthiness, being part of the less valued groups. But it isn't just that vulnerability arises, it is actually engendered in the less powerful by the more powerful. And then people are shamed for showing signs of vulnerability: girls are shamed for being "selfish" or too needy, while boys are shamed for being fearful or dependent; women on welfare are shamed for needing assistance; women are shamed for wanting relationships too much. People of color are shamed, gays and lesbians are shamed, people with physical challenges are shamed, people without money are shamed, older people and people who are sick are shamed. The dominant system isolates and silences with this shaming, and thus subverts challenges to its power and avoids conflict from subordinate groups. If we are unable to stay with the vulnerability of shame, both in and out of therapy, it can also lead to serious disconnections.

When we are struggling to be certain and invulnerable ("strong") we become less open, less ready to listen responsively, more rigid and dogmatic. Looking for certainty in therapy can lead to disempowerment for both client and therapist. Some of my most unhelpful therapy sessions occur when I am feeling a need to know, usually inspired by fear or helplessness or my shame about not being a "good enough therapist." My need to be the expert, to know, often bypasses the resources of the client. Relational-Cultural Therapy depends on responsiveness, mutual curiosity, and courage–it is a dialogue. The not knowing, the questions, are always at the center.

I think I've always been asking the unanswerable questions: what is life about, what is the meaning of all this? It's something I can't quite control in myself despite my knowledge that there isn't any answer, that, as Rilke (1934) says, we live the question. But I keep probing these issues with people, just as I keep pestering people with the question, "What makes for change in life, in therapy, in relationships?" My older sister, very aware of this tendency of mine that she's been dealing with since I was probably five years old, recently sent me a note pad that said, "What if the hokey pokey *is* what it's all about?" At its best, I think life is about learning and loving. I think movement and change is the natural order of things, that seeking connection is part of that order. I think things get "stuck" when we disconnect, when we move out of connection, when we claim too much for the self, when we fail to allow vulnerability, when we stop learning, and when we feel we have to have the answers. The questions for therapy, and perhaps for the larger picture of social change, are about how we can resist the forces of disconnection that impede the movement and change that connection creates. Connection is a powerful force for change.

LOVE

I want to end by speaking briefly about love. I feel vulnerable about doing this and I had actually written some of this before the last Harvard conference and then omitted it at the last minute. Love as a healing force is spoken of so little in therapeutic literature. I see a lot of therapists in my practice. A frequent comment I hear about their clients is, "I just love her," said with directness, lack of discomfort, and a good deal of clarity and feeling. I also hear, "She's driving me crazy," etc., but in the love statement the affect is direct, unself-conscious, and certainly resonates with the way I feel about the people I see in my practice. But I was thinking about how infrequently I have heard this kind of love spoken of in textbooks, case conferences, and supervision groups. Why is love, as part of the therapeutic relationship, part of the healing, spoken of so little in therapeutic literature, or in therapy itself? And, is love different from the desire to participate in growth-fostering connection? I would suggest that somehow the dominant culture's emphasis on power and control has eclipsed our appreciation of love in healing and creating change. Intellectual insight and making unconscious conflict conscious have overshadowed the important work of connecting and creating growth-fostering relationships. In a patriarchal "power over" culture love gets narrowed to romantic, sexualized, and usually heterosexual relationships, which are themselves constructions of power imbalance. It becomes preempted and trivialized.

I myself get caught in this. For instance, when a client asked (not long ago enough for me to blame my response on youth or inexperience), "Do you love me?" I became anxious, imagining all the misconstruals, sexual, romantic, and otherwise, that might occur. I responded cautiously (and some of my cautiousness was appropriate), "Of course I care about you." At least I didn't do the "what makes you ask?" number. The question is not so surprising: Who doesn't want to know if they are loved, in therapy or elsewhere? She persisted, "But do you *love* me?" Then I went into a long discourse on what I think love is and isn't. I talked about the different kinds of love: friendly love, motherly love, romantic love, sexual love, agape, platonic love, lunatic love, unconditional love, empathic attunement, and on and on, using all the intellectualizing disconnections I could find. My client finally exclaimed in the middle of one of these, "All right I see this makes you anxious. I'll settle for your word *care*. You care about me."

How different it was for Irene Stiver in addressing her clients at the end of her life! After Irene realized she would be unable to resume her clinical practice because of her illness, she asked Pam Peck and me to compose a letter to her clients. She wanted to let them know how sorry she was not to be able to say goodbye in person, and to convey her caring about them. Writing the letter was a very difficult assignment. Pam and I worked hard on the letter; and we came up with something that felt caring, respectful, sad, and appreciative. But when we read it to Irene, she said, "Well you've left out the most important thing. I've got to speak about the love." She then dictated the following: "It has become even clearer to me that love is what it's all about. Not only at this time, but also throughout our relationship, I have felt your love and deep caring for me. In turn, I hope that you feel my love for you. My hope is that you will hold onto this love and build on it in your life. Thank you for the privilege of being part of your life."

Love is a state of vulnerability. In loving, we are affected strongly by the other person and we share that effect. We are also affecting the other person in deep ways. bell hooks (2000) wrote, "The mutual practice of giving and receiving is an everyday ritual when we know true love. A generous heart is always open, always ready to receive our coming and going. In the midst of such love we need never fear abandonment. This is the most precious gift that love offers, the experience of knowing we always belong" (p. 164). I would add, we know that we matter, that the other matters, and that there is mutual responsiveness. We know that relationships matter. This takes us out of the narrow confines of the separate-self trying to assert its worth in autonomy and independence.

Love is ultimately about vulnerability, courage, and growth. Growth-fostering relationships are to my mind essentially loving relationships that connect us to one another and to ourselves. We open ourselves to vulnerability, we allow people to have an impact on us, we let people see that they matter; we care deeply about their growth and well-being. The concept of mutuality is easier for me to talk about in therapy than love, given the complicated baggage that the word love carries. But I think we should begin to reclaim the language of love, away from the sexualized, romanticized distortions of the dominant culture, and bring it back into the heart of caring and healing. Perhaps the language of love is the real antidote to the language of power-over others. bell hooks (2000) also wrote, "We can collectively regain our faith in the transformative power of love by cultivating courage, the strength to stand up for what we believe in, to be accountable both in work and deed" (p. 92). And Thomas Merton (1979) concluded, "We don't become fully human until we give ourselves to each other in love" (p. 27). In love, we transcend separateness, we extend ourselves to others, we find ways to navigate conflict, we see that vulnerability is necessary to growth, and we move toward increasing mutual connection.

REFERENCES

Collins, P. H. (2000). *Black feminist thought knowledge, consciousness, and the politics of empowerment* (Rev. 10th anniversary ed., 2nd ed.). New York: Routledge.

Cushman, P. (1995). *Constructing the self, constructing America: A cultural history of psychotherapy.* Boston, MA: Addison-Wesley Pub.

Gilligan, C., Rogers, A. G., & Tolman, D. L. (Eds.). (1991). *Women, girls, and psychotherapy: Reframing resistance.* New York: Harrington Park Press.

hooks, b. (2000). *All about love: New visions.* New York: William Morrow.

Jordan, J. (1981). *Civil wars.* Boston: Beacon Press.

Jordan, J. V. (1989). Relational development: Therapeutic implications of empathy and shame. *Work in Progress, No. 39.* Wellesley, MA: Stone Center Working Paper Series.

Jordan, J. V. (1990). Courage in connection: Conflict, compassion, creativity. *Work in Progress, No. 45.* Wellesley, MA: Stone Center Working Paper Series.

Jordan, J. V. (1992a). Relational resilience. *Work in Progress, No. 57.* Wellesley, MA: Stone Center Working Paper Series.

Jordan, J. V. (1992b). The relational self: A new perspective for understanding women's development. *Contemporary Psychotherapy Review, 1,* 56-71.

Jordan, J. V. (1996). Boundaries: A relational perspective. *Psychotherapy Forum, 1*(2), 4-5.

Jordan, J. V. (1999). Toward connection and competence. *Work in Progress No. 83.* Wellesley, MA: Stone Center Working Paper Series.

Jordan, J. V. (2001). A relational-cultural model: Healing through mutual empathy. *Bulletin of the Menninger Clinic, 65*(1), 92-103.

Lawrence-Lightfoot, S. (1999). *Respect: An exploration.* Reading, MA. Perseus Books.

McIntosh, P. (1988). White privilege and male privilege: A personal account of coming to see correspondences through work in women's studies. *Working Paper, No. 189.* Wellesley, MA: Center for Research on Women.

Merton, T. (1979). *Love and living.* (N. Burton Stone, & P. Hart, Eds.). New York: Farrar, Straus, and Giroux.

Miller, J. B. (1986). What do we mean by relationships? *Work in Progress, No. 22.* Wellesley, MA: Stone Center Working Paper Series.

Miller, J. B., &, Stiver, I. P. (1997). *The healing connection: How women form relationships in therapy and in life.* Boston, MA: Beacon Press.

Miller, J. B., Jordan, J. V., Stiver, I. P., Surrey, J., Walker, M., & Eldridge, N. (1999). Therapists' authenticity. *Work in Progress No. 82.* Wellesley, MA: Stone Center Working Paper Series.

Oxford English Dictionary. (compacted). (1971). Oxford: Clarendon Press.

Rilke, R. M. (2001). *Letters to a young poet.* (M.D. Herter Norton, Trans.). New York: Modern Library. (Original work published 1934).

Taylor, S. E. (2002). *The tending instinct: How nurturing is essential to who we are and how we live.* New York: Times Books.

Taylor, S. E., Cousino Klein, L., Gruenewald, T. L., Guring, R. A. R., Lewis, B. P., & Upgdegraff, J. A. (2000). Behavioral responses to stress in females: Tend-andbefriend, not fight-or-flight. *Psychological Review, 107*(3), 411-429.

Ward, J. V. (2000). *The skin we're in: Teaching our children to be emotionally strong, socially smart, spiritually connected.* New York: Free Press.

Commitment to Connection in a Culture of Fear

Judith V. Jordan

SUMMARY. This article was originally presented at the May 2004 *Learning from Women Conference* sponsored by Harvard Medical School and the Jean Baker Miller Training Institute. It examines the ways in which cultural and personal denial of fear and vulnerability contribute to a sense of isolation. Fear is manipulated in hierarchical settings to ensure the preservation of existing power arrangements. In a culture built on exploitation of fear, people do not experience the safety necessary to let their inevitable vulnerabilities show. Unmitigated chronic fear is an unsafe context that leads to a traumatic sense of disempowerment and personal immobilization, whether it is in war, childhood sexual abuse, living with a battering partner, or, perhaps in a more subtle way, in being immersed in massages of un-safety, danger, and having no influence in the larger public domain. Through mutual empathy we can heal these places of fear and disconnection. Mutual empathy arises in a context of profound respect, authentic responsiveness, humility, non-defensiveness, an attitude of curiosity, mindfulness (staying with the "not knowing"), and an appreciation of the power of learning. Movement out of isolation helps us pass through fear to hope and ultimately leads to growth and more connection.

Judith V. Jordan, PhD, is Founding Scholar and Director of the Jean Baker Miller Training Institute and Co-Director of Working Connections Project; Assistant Professor, Harvard Medical School; co-author of *Women's Growth in Connection*; editor of *Women's Growth in Diversity*; and co-editor of *The Complexity of Connection*, JBMTI.

INTRODUCTION

Fear is often a useful and, at times, a lifesaving affective signal. It is also the ultimate reminder of our vulnerability. Fear moves us to escape from danger. At its best, in the right context, it moves us to seek safety in connection. In a culture or situation that supports vulnerability, fear leads us toward engagement; we turn to others for help and comfort. At a core level we all know our ultimate dependence on one another, and we live with awareness of our own mortality and the mortality of those we love. The deepest and most abiding human fear may be the fear of disconnection and isolation.

Some have called our current era the "age of anxiety," with over 50 million people in this country suffering from various anxiety disorders. American culture has been specifically referred to as the most anxious, frightened society in history (Shaw, 1994). While fear, vulnerability, and emotional suffering are inevitable aspects of life, the experience of fear is distorted when connections are not safe, when vulnerability is not supported, and fear is denied or viewed as a sign of weakness and unworthiness. Furthermore, fear is often stimulated by those in power as a way to disempower and exercise social control over others. In fact, fear is the cornerstone of "power-over systems." "Directing fear in a society is tantamount to controlling that society" (Altheide, 2002, p. 17). Today we are witnessing the way the dominant-ruling group fuels people's fears: about weapons of mass destruction, about Iraq, about our personal safety in the face of anthrax, about the dangers of gay marriage and gay families, to name a few. A recent full-page ad in the *Boston Globe* pointed to very selective and erroneous "scientific evidence" documenting the destructiveness of same-sex parenting. This was clearly aimed at showing that not only children, but also the "good life" as we know it (i.e., patriarchal marriage) would be destroyed by the deviance of same-sex loving couples daring to establish families. We can learn much about a society by the way it addresses fear and vulnerability. Are vulnerable and "different" populations punished as weak "losers?" Are they possibly viewed as dangerous subverters of the status quo? Or are they seen as those whose disadvantage is to be responded to with compassion and care? And might they be seen as those whose difference could provide creative energy for the whole society? Is power used to control and subjugate or to empower and encourage?

Our culture endlessly amplifies fear. We live in a culture of violence, and we are exposed to it daily. The media stimulates our fear, then advertisers step in to offer relief. There is well-publicized crime against children from strangers, although the more hidden dangers from their nuclear families are made less public. We know that women are least safe in their own kitchens and bedrooms where partner abuse and murder occur at an alarming rate (so much for the success of the patriarchal family!). Aggressive solutions to international problems are undertaken with little apparent regard for the devastating human consequences of war and military invasion. Terrorism, a horrible disruptive process whose real aim is the creation of destabilizing, unremitting fear, can send us not just to our places of vulnerability, but to a defensive preoccupation with being invulnerable, or safe in armed isolation.

Lest we think that a climate of fear is an unintended outcome in systems based on establishing dominance, I'd like to suggest that the creation of fear is central to establishing control over others. In a book called *The Peculiar Institution* (Stamp,1989) about American slavery, a slave master is quoted as giving the following prescription for the management of slaves:

1. Establish and maintain strict discipline.
2. Implant in the bondsmen themselves a consciousness of personal inferiority.
3. Awe them with a sense of their master's enormous power.
4. Persuade the bondsmen to take an interest in the master's enterprise.
5. Impress the slaves with their helplessness, to create in them a habit of perfect dependence upon their masters.

A Charlestonian slave master added that the only principle upon which slavery could be maintained was "the principle of fear," or as a North Carolina mistress noted, "make them stand in fear" (p. 146). Fear is not an accidental consequence of institutions that exercise power over others; it is the driving force that deepens and expands the power and the potential for abuse. Fear is first created *within* the non-dominant groups in order to control them, and then fear *of* the non-dominant groups is created within the dominant group to rationalize their control over the non-dominants. It is an insidious, double-edged sword meant to buttress the power of those at the top.

In more subtle ways, creation of fear plays out in patriarchal white families, hierarchical corporations, and schools. Seventy-six percent of students in a Midwestern study said they have been bullied and 14% had severe reactions. Everyday 160,000 children miss school due to fear of attack or intimidation (Fried & Fried, 1996). The 1993 American Association of University Women study, *Hostile Hallways*, indicates that "85% of girls and 76% of boys reported being sexually harassed at some point in school" (p. 60).

Shame, disrespect, and humiliation all are based on fear. Vulnerability is vigorously shamed in our culture and humiliation often involves enforced and exposed vulnerability. Categorical disrespect or prejudice, the dismissal of a person based on stereotype, is a frightening process of dehumanization and fear-induction. There is ample evidence from developmental studies that people's immediate response to fear is to reach out for a caring other (Taylor, 2002). We also reach out to care for others who are in distress. While early attachment theorists would suggest that this movement toward others naturally declines as the child internalizes maternal function, there is accumulating evidence that this reaching out to engage in times of fear and stress is a lifelong pattern if it is not curtailed by socialization practices which make turning to others a sign of weakness.

DENIAL OF FEAR

While North American 21st Century dominant culture generates and feeds on the fears of the less powerful, it is also heavily invested in the denial of fear, the denial of our need for connection, and the manipulation of fear for sociopolitical/economic reasons. In the socialization of boys especially, signs of vulnerability and fear are severely punished. In fact, adolescent boys die in alarming numbers in car accidents and daredevil feats as they are determined to demonstrate the absence of fear. To be fearful is to be "a girl," a wimp. A woman came up to me at the end of a presentation I gave on raising boys and girls. She said, "I'm a feminist, I've raised my boys with feminist values. My 8-year-old son was on a mostly boys' soccer team. There was one girl on this team, who was an exceptionally skilled player. At one of the breaks, a boy from the other team came up to my son and taunted him. 'You're on a girls' team, you're a girl–you're just girls.'" The mother said her son looked upset, hurt, and angry and struggled with a response. Eventually her son countered with, "We are *not* girls. We're *not* girls." Then he paused and a change came over his face. "We're *not* girls. We're–WOMEN!!" One of the primary rites of passage into manhood for American boys is defiance of fear. As Miriam Greenspan (2003) noted, "the culture of patriarchy punishes fearful men and fearless women" (p. 182). In the film *Iron Jawed Angels* (2004) about Alice Paul, a little-celebrated suffragette who led a hunger strike in support of women getting the vote, a psychiatrist who was called in to document Paul's insanity refused to do so, noting, "Courageous women are often called insane."

Vulnerability defines our humanity. Fear signals our vulnerability. Denial of fear and vulnerability creates our most profound alienation from others and ourselves and generates our worst isolation. The answer to vulnerability and fear is not denial, greater development of unilateral power and dominance, or stockpiling of emotional or material weapons. Rather it is through connecting and establishing a sense of meaning that involves transcending the separate self. My sister said to me recently (half in jest but half seriously I think), "I feel like I'm here to serve others but sometimes I wonder what the others are here for?" According to Robert Putnam (2000) who wrote *Bowling Alone*, "Americans have become steadily more disconnected from one another and from public and private institutions over the course of the last 25 or 30 years" (p. 26).

An ethic of "self-interest" prevails in Western psychology. We have compulsively focused on the self and its ability to achieve. We have been led to believe that self-interest is healthy and is to be encouraged, and that lack of self-interest is a sign of pathology. As Dale Miller (1999) points out:

> The psychological theory of self-interest becomes a self-fulfilling prophecy. Self-interest is not simply an abstract theoretical concept but a collectively shared ideology. The theory of self-interest has spawned a norm of self-interest, the consequence of which is that people often act and speak in accordance with their perceived self-interest solely because they believe to-do otherwise is to violate a powerful descriptive and prescriptive expectation. (p. 1053-4)

Contrary to much psychological theory which posits that infants are born greedy and aggressive and alone ("You're born alone, you die alone"... no mother made that one up!!!), we at the *Jean Baker Miller Training Institute* believe that self-interest and primary aggression are no more basically human than the desire for connection and the capacity to love. *The Seville Statement on Violence* (Dalai Lama & Cutler, 1998), made by 20 top scientists from around the world, noted:

> It is scientifically incorrect to say that we have an inherited tendency to make war or act violent. That behavior is not genetically programmed into human nature. We have the potential to develop into gentle caring people or violent aggressive people; the impulse that gets emphasized is largely a matter of training. (p. 58)

Data on giving and volunteer work (Luks, 1992) indicates that giving to others–participating in generative activity with others–increases our sense of well-being and our physical health. Mutual interest serves all of us; self-interest does not.

The psychological concept of the "separate self" has been constructed largely in a white, middle-class, heterosexual, capitalistic culture. It is totally identified with a model of "power over." A separate-self model is predicated on a spatial metaphor (remember, "self" is a metaphor, not reality) that involves a bounded entity seeking protection by building better boundaries against an impinging environment or by accruing power over others. To be influenced by another is potentially dangerous in this system.

But being separate also generates fear. In this system, then, individuals should get everything from the outside to the inside as fast and securely as they can–that includes building solid intrapsychic structure. This model supports and creates the basis for a solidly consuming culture. One must buy a new cosmetic, buy a new car, drink more, and eat more to feel better. We live with a deep irony at the heart of this system: Under the pressure to be totally independent and separate, which is impossible, we are manipulated into created dependencies that give more economic power to those in power. Therefore, those who build the best boundaries, who are the least influenced by others, and who gather the most material stuff are seen as successful and powerful. But nobody ever really makes it to this state of total independence and success, even though they wish to project the image that they have–not even the white, middle-class, privileged men who were "born on third base and thought they hit a triple."

Plain and simple, we need to connect to survive and thrive. Correlations between social connectedness and positive child development are robustly high (Putnam, 2000). Studies have shown that during adolescence, one good relationship with an adult is the best protection against high-risk behaviors of suicidality, violence, and substance abuse (Resnick, 1997).

Because connection is so basic to our well-being, I would like to suggest that fear of isolation is probably the most profound fear that human beings experience. Ironically, this knowledge is used in our prisons where isolation or solitary confinement is the most awful punishment, aside from death, that we can imagine. Bowlby (1973) noted that separation and interpersonal loss are at the very roots of the human experiences of fear, sadness, and sorrow. But instead of celebrating our need for connection and building a society that supports that need, we have created the illusion of the separate self.

THE RELATIONAL-CULTURAL MODEL

The Relational-Cultural Model of the Stone Center posits that connection is at the core of human growth and development. Isolation is seen as the primary source of human suffering. The path of human development is through movement to increasingly differentiated and growth-fostering connection. Chronic disconnections are most destructive when they result from the non-responsiveness or violations from important and powerful people in our lives. When we are hurt, misunderstood, or violated in some way, we may attempt to represent our experience to the injuring person. But if we are not responded to, we learn to suppress our experience and disconnect from both our own feelings and the other person. If, on the other hand, we are able to express our feelings and the other person responds with care–showing that we have had an effect–then we feel that we are effective in the relationship, that we matter, and that we can participate in creating a growth-fostering and healthy relationship.

The Relational-Cultural Model cares about suffering incurred at the individual level but we also care about the effects of disconnection at a societal level (Walker, 1999), in particular, the ways that power differentials, forces of stratification, privilege, and marginalization can disconnect and disempower individuals and groups of people. In this model it is essential that we look at context and that we do not assume that the person–or group–presenting with pain *is* the problem. We need to ask, "Where is the pain?" and "Where is the problem?" They often arise in different places. We should always remember that part of the work of a dominant group is to get the subjugated or non-dominant group to internalize the following construction: "I am the problem because I feel the pain."

As Maureen Walker (2004) has pointed out, theories about human development must answer the questions, "What purpose and whose interest does the theory serve?" A similar sentiment is expressed in the African proverb, "Until the lions have their historians, all tales of hunting will glorify the hunter" (Dalai Lama & Cutler, 1998, p. 87). The separate-self model serves a competitive, consuming, and mobile culture. The hunter still tells the tale.

While this may seem like a large leap, I'd like to move from the macro to the micro, because these social forces converge on people and very explicitly affect the biological and psychological functioning of the individual which ultimately affects the capacity to engage in community. Fear has an impact on our feelings, on our neurochemistry, and on our brains individually and collectively (Banks, 2001). I'd like to begin to show how connection has a positive and healing effect on our feelings, neurochemistry, brains, and ultimately on our ability to make use of connection and community to dissipate fear.

THE NEUROBIOLOGY OF FEAR, DISCONNECTION, AND CONNECTION

When we are afraid or stressed, our hearts race, our blood pressure goes up, and our epinephrine and norepinephrine surge. Our sympathetic nervous system is activated so that we are ready to take action. Countering this arousal, the hormone oxytocin often creates a calming effect, leading animals and people to seek more contact when they are stressed or afraid, thus reducing the "fight or flight" response. This is at the heart of the "tend and befriend" response observed in females under stress, delineated by Shelly Taylor and her colleagues (2002). Interestingly, oxytocin is enhanced by estrogen and suppressed by the male stress hormones (like vasopressin) and thus the "fight or flight response" is not modulated in males in the same way it is in females. Males and females may experience fear differently by virtue of both nature *and* nurture.

What constitutes stress and pain and what leads to fear in an organism has also been clarified in a groundbreaking study reported on this past year by Eisenberger and Lieberman (2003). These researchers have discovered that social pain and physical pain share parts of the same underlying brain processing system, and they suggest that "social connection is a need as basic as air, water, or food and that like the more traditional needs, the absence of social connection causes pain" (p. 2). They note that we are actually "hard wired" to experience distress upon separation and comfort upon reunion.

Social pain can be defined as "distressing experience arising from the perception of psychological distance from close others or from the social group" (p. 7). Anticipating social pain creates fear. Although attachment theorists have studied something like this for years in their separation studies, what is becoming clearer is that social pain–pain around separation and exclusion–persists throughout the lifespan. Being someone who has suffered from so-called "separation anxiety" my whole life and having been pathologized for it, I welcome these new normalizing data with special warmth and relief. These researchers conclude:

> We are beginning to appreciate that the need for social connection is so essential to survival, at least in mammalian species that being left out or disconnected from the social group is processed by the brain in a manner similar to physical pain. (p. 36)

Perceiving that one is not valued in a relationship literally leads to "hurt feelings" and real pain, registered in the anterior cingulate cortex. The authors comment:

> One very tangible consequence of assuming that social pain is not as valid or legitimate as physical pain is a societal acceptance of certain elicitors of social pain, such as prejudice and racism. (p. 37)

These are profoundly important empirical findings that support the work in which the Stone Center has been engaged for 25 years. Connections matter, individual isolation matters, and social pain and marginalization matter.

In a report from the Commission on Children at Risk in 2003 entitled, *Hardwired to Connect*, distinguished researchers from around the country concluded that "we are born to form attachments, that our brains are physically wired to develop in tandem with another's through emotional communication, beginning before words are spoken" (p. 16). They also concluded that we are hardwired for meaning: "born with a built-in capacity and drive to search for purpose and reflect on life's ultimate ends" (p. 14).

Allan Schore (2003), who has also been exploring the psychobiology of attachment in the mother-infant dyad, notes that mutuality enhances the development of the right prefrontal cortex in both mother and child. This is the part of the brain, which mediates empathic cognition and perception of emotional states, and modulates amygdala functions. Mutual responsiveness actually creates growth in this essential part of the brain and interruption of mutuality interferes with its development. In the mother-child relationship–just as in therapy–how we respond to acute disconnections determines either resilience or movement into chronic disconnection. Chronic disconnection literally alters brain structure, which in turn leads to more disconnection. We now have evidence at the neurobiological level of the power of connection, of the destructiveness of chronic disconnection, and of how essential mutuality is to our well-being.

While ordinary failures of mutuality constitute usual and expectable events in relationships, the result of chronic and severe relational trauma is what Perry called "fear-terror" (Schore, 2003, p. 247). When an infant or child is sexually, physically, or emotionally abused by a caregiver, an intolerable fear situation arises; the child is alarmed by the caregiver, but the child cannot approach the caregiver for comfort since the caregiver is also the source of fear. When abuse is chronic, there is a situation of immobilizing fear–protective disconnection as well as guarded, inauthentic responses become the rule. Empathic responsiveness and mutual empathy provide opportunities for a return to mutuality. In these corrective interactions, mutual synchronization of the prefrontal cortex occurs, which ultimately lessens fear, isolation, and the feeling of "not mattering." At the neurobiological level, empathic attunement and good connection generate change in the ability to connect for both people. Therapy provides a wonderful relational opportunity to rework the neurological and psychological consequences of failed connection. This is not re-parenting, but it does in fact involve a reworking of the neurological circuits and psychological meaning-making. In a way psychotherapy can provide what bell hooks (1989) describes as a "site of radical openness," where real change can happen and where connection can begin to undo the damage of stress and fear.

THERAPY

Studies of therapy have indicated that most of the variance in therapy outcome studies can be accounted for by relationship factors. A study by Najavits and Strupp in 1994 indicated that the "basic capacities of human relating–warmth, affirmation, and a minimum of attack and blame–may be at the center of effective psychotherapeutic intervention" (Norcross, 2002, p. 24). The psychotherapy relationship is about: creating change; slowly and carefully finding flexibility where there was rigidity; creating the courage to move into vulnerability where protective disconnection and closing down prevailed; finding the possibility of new connections and new understandings of old connections; and creating relational hope where there had been fear and despair–that awful sense of "I'm all alone and I can't make a difference." This process is based on mutual empathy and mutual responsiveness, which allow greater authenticity and greater connection with one's inner experience, as well as with the other person. The way we work with disconnections, ruptures, and empathic failures may be *the* most crucial factor to consider in understanding how change and healing happens in therapy. Psychotherapy is a place of *relational possibility*. As one client noted, "Fear determines my places of disconnection. If I can't get beyond the fear, I'm stuck." In therapy the work *is* to stay present with the feelings and to move with the client through the times of disconnection, particularly when we, as therapists, have contributed to the rupture. It sounds easy, but it is not.

Relational-Cultural Therapy is about healing through connection–about being moved and changed in relationship. The dogma of traditional therapy is that the therapist should "not be moved," or more specifically should not be openly responsive. Allowing the client to see that he or she has had an impact on the therapist is seen as threatening the client's sense of safety and the neutrality necessary to develop and work on transference phenomenon. While "blank screen" prescriptions are rarely given anymore, they hover in the background in most traditional therapies where it is often suggested that engagement–being seen and known as an emotionally present person–will be unsafe and destructive for the client. Relational-Cultural Theory (RCT) suggests the opposite is true: Real mutual responsiveness and engagement is necessary for healing. And I believe that our most recent discoveries in neurobiology support these suggested shifts in approach. The therapist's affective presence, mediated by clinical judgment, is essential to the movement of therapy. Affective presence means that the therapist must be open to being affected by the client and that the client in turn will be affected by the therapist's affect. This is mutual empathy. It creates more nuanced and elaborated affects and cognitions, and lessens isolation and the fear that accompanies it.

The culture of traditional psychotherapy inevitably reflects the culture of the dominant group, which often values logic, certainty, linear development toward separateness, as well as top-down learning, objectivity, and instrumentality. The tradition of interpretation invites the illusion of certain and oracular knowledge. Rosanne Adams commented at last year's Summer Training Institute (personal communication, June, 2003), "The supply of interpretations far exceeds the demand." Who as a client really wants an interpretation and how often do interpretations feel resonant and validating? In these traditional systems the therapist is opaque and mystified–only the client is self-revealing and the revelations increase his or her vulnerability. I am not advocating an abundance of factual self-disclosures on the part of the therapist. The therapist's responsiveness must be guided by anticipatory empathy, which is an awareness of the possible impact of our interventions on the client.

The work of the therapist in dealing with the inevitable fear that brings people to therapy is to establish a safe-enough context in which to address the fear. Therapists have differing ideas about how that safety is best achieved. I believe that for the therapist to be a "safe enough" person, she must be clear about her responsiveness and clear about the limits of her ability to respond. For the most terrified of our clients, sexual and physical abuse survivors, a power-over, authoritarian attitude and opaque stance on the part of the therapist can only be triggering and re-traumatizing, even when imposed with the most benign of intentions. Being in relationship with powerful others does not create a sense of possibility or safety for an abuse survivor; it exacerbates fear and terror. Furthermore, when met with neutrality, perhaps similar to what infant researchers have called "still-face" (Tronick & Weinberg, 1997) these clients may move into frantic, fear-driven efforts to find responsiveness. This often leads to more disconnection.

In therapy we look for the place of *relational possibility*. When clients close down, complexity is reduced, and in increasing rigidity they resort to old, well-worn and over-generalized images and coping strategies. People are often emotionally triggered and amygdala reactivity takes over. Relational images are those expectations for relationship that we carry with us from the past into our present lives (Miller & Stiver, 1997). The ones that give us trouble, negative relational images, are those that arise from nonresponsive or hurtful interactions with important and powerful early figures. Breaking free of or modifying old, fixed, negative relational images allows new relational possibilities. Thus, where there was pathological certainty and inflexibility in the client's relational expectations, therapists help create healthy uncertainty, flexibility, and appreciation of complexity. We support the growth of new relational images. We do this through the use of mutual empathy and working with discrepant relational images. Discrepant relational images are those images and expectations that are at odds with the primary organizing images a person carries. They are often sites of hope and possibility.

SUE'S STORY

Sue is a young woman who grew up in a household that was riddled with psychosis and violence. She witnessed frequent beatings of her mother by her father. Her mother had been hospitalized psychiatrically often, and under traumatic conditions (against her will, by policemen). She would sometimes awaken the children in the middle of the night to walk some distance to "meet with Jesus." Sue and her sister had also experienced sexual and physical abuse. At the age of six, in a moment of bravado, Sue climbed a very high tree in her back yard, and when she reached about two stories up, she suddenly realized where she was and she froze, unable to move up or down, wailing uncontrollably. Her mother stood at the bottom of the tree also wailing helplessly. It took an alert neighbor to call the fire department, who dispatched an engine with a long ladder to help Sue get down. But aside from when she was stuck up in the tree, Sue had rarely noticed as a child, or even in retrospect, how frightened she usually was, what a terrifying world she lived in. She was mostly numb, in denial of her fear. It was not safe enough for her to feel her fear. This image of being stuck up in the tree fit one of her dominant relational images of "I'm in danger and alone, and if I ask for help, I throw others into distress." Unlike most of the time when she was in danger and didn't feel it, in this memory she was aware of and experienced her fear. Over time this image became a focal point for reconnecting with her real experience of fear and slowly finding a way through it.

Sue's core relational image could be summarized as "If I am myself and really authentic, others abandon me or hate me." As a child, whenever she had tried to state her needs, protect herself, or stand up for her sister, the adults around her hurt her. But then there was Mrs. Richards, her fifth grade teacher, who saw Sue's intelligence and vulnerability and encouraged her creative, questioning spirit. Mrs. Richards loved Sue's "out of the box" thinking and her willingness to take intellectual chances. For Sue the discrepant relational image in this case was "when I am curious and am being myself, I am responded to with warmth and love and respect." While this image was almost exclusively limited to her relationship with Mrs. Richards, this small spark of positive energy later became the place for relational possibility and hope.

It was in her first year at college that things unraveled for Sue. She began to cut herself, spend days in bed, and feel suicidal. She was sent to a psychiatric hospital where she had the good fortune to be treated by a courageous and creative psychology intern for one year. The hope given to her long ago by Mrs. Richards was rekindled. But as she began to open up to this therapist and also began to feel attached to her, the flood gates of fear began to open up as well. She needed to call the therapist frequently, she sometimes could not talk at all in sessions, and she could not leave the therapist's office at the end of sessions. She continued to be self-destructive. Unfortunately the intern–this incredibly warm, patient, and kind woman–left the area at the end of her internship. Following this, Sue floated from one therapist to another; she fired this one, one stopped working with her because she wouldn't contract for safety, and so it went.

Knowing I had been her intern's supervisor, Sue called me after several years and in a weak–or possibly courageous and wise–moment, I agreed to see her. Sue taught me many lessons in our several years of working together. I lost more sleep over her than anyone else I ever worked with. I worried more, and in fact I learned more about fear than I ever wanted to know. I screwed up more, felt more doubt and shame about my incompetence, and truth be told, I probably grew more. Once, when I was firmly stating my limits of what I could or couldn't do in terms of experiencing fear with her, she said quite clearly, "You need to be up in that tree with me. You need to know my fear." She was right that I needed to be with her, but I also needed to help both of us be anchored in a safe enough place. I said, "Sue, if I'm up in that tree with you, as a scared and frozen six-year old, I can't be of help. I've got to be on the fire ladder holding on to you and to something solid below so we can both get down. I can taste your fear but I can't be completely in it with you." It took a while for that approach to work for both of us. I often felt we were both up that tree with no back-up ladders or other people, and that I was being asked to hold hope when my fear led me only to a wish to control the situation. Sometimes I simply felt a powerful impulse to disconnect. I remember once saying to her about a different issue, in what I thought was great empathy, "You must be so scared," and she looked at me and with great clarity said, "No, Judy, you're so scared." And she was right. She helped me come back into the uncertainty we were in together–scared but now more present.

Bessel Van der Kolk (1987) once stated that Post-Traumatic Stress Disorder is a disorder of hope. In many ways all problems involving relational failures or violations generate disorders of hope. Empathy and compassion are essential to the rebuilding of hope. The Latin root of the word emotion is *mo teri*, to move. Feelings move us–they're meant to move us!! Fear is meant to move us. Hope, like courage, is built in relationship, not in isolation, and it makes movement possible. How can we, therapists and clients alike, use our fear to move back into reparative connection, toward courage and resilience?

The *quality of presence* we bring to therapeutic relationships is very important. It involves *profound*, even radical, *respect* and a deep openness to being affected. In the powerful documentary, *The Color of Fear* (1994), an eloquent African American man angrily says to a clueless white man, "You have to be willing to be changed by my experience as I am by yours." This is the essence of mutual respect. It is about valuing our clients, valuing their strengths, their wisdom, their suffering, their struggles, really seeing things through their experience, and being responsive to their feelings.

As therapists we need to be appropriately aware of our limitations and strengths. I am not a "relational expert"; ask anyone who knows me. I struggle in concrete and sometimes embarrassing ways to build relationships. I joke sometimes about a first appointment with a client where she said to me "If you really knew me you wouldn't want to work with me." And I thought to myself, "If you really knew *me* you wouldn't want to work with me." In part, humility can contribute to non-defensiveness and this involves not getting caught in protecting our own *images* of ourselves. It is important to protect our relationships and ourselves but protecting our *images* of ourselves usually moves us out of relationship. We need to practice with an attitude of curiosity and mindfulness, particularly staying with the "not knowing" and the complexity of relating. Together we build faith in our relationships, based on our particular history of negotiating conflict, uncertainty, and disconnections. I have often used the image of the therapist "holding the umbrella of connection," over all the misattunements, injuries, disappointments, and conflicts that are part of the fabric of all relationships.

Having put forth all these idealistic intentions of practicing from a relational point of view, let me add, I give advice too often, I philosophize, I laugh and joke with clients, I worry too much about people and still lose sleep at times when they are in crisis, I teach people to meditate, I refer people to Eye Movement Desensitization and Reprocessing and Cognitive Behavioral Therapy, and people terminate with me and go on to do wonderful work with other therapists. I get distracted by papers I'm trying to write while I'm sitting with people, I've pinched myself to stay awake on occasion, I've taken gifts, I've refused gifts, and, on occasion, I've even given gifts. I still think Irene or Jean would be doing a better job than I am (maybe you'll think so too now). I'm grateful that Jean has recently spoken about the importance of being wrong. I think admitting one's limitations, apologizing, moving into humility, and tolerating uncertainty are essential to providing growing spaces for all of us. Furthermore, it is important to share with our experiences of more intense vulnerability in our work with trusted colleagues.

Here's a simplistic one sentence synopsis of what I think might help us in our therapy work and in our lives: We need to practice compassion, curiosity, and courage while we tolerate complexity, conflict, and confusion in a spirit of shared humanity, humor, and humility.

CLOSING COMMENTS

I want to conclude on a quirky note of optimism. The April 13, 2004 *New York Times* carried the following story: "No Time for Bullies: Baboons Retool Their Culture," by Natalie Angier. Apparently 20 years ago a troop of Savanna baboons in Kenya experienced an outbreak of tuberculosis that "killed off the biggest, nastiest, and most despotic males, setting the stage for a social and behavioral transformation unlike any seen in this notoriously truculent primate." The dead were all dominant adult males that had beaten out another baboon troop to get at meat in a garbage dump that was contaminated with bovine tuberculosis. "Left behind in the troop, designated the Forest Troop, were the 50 percent of the males that had been too subordinate to try dump brawling as well as the females and their young." What followed was a complete change in the baboon culture: The hierarchy relaxed and the baboons began to "use affection and mutual grooming, rather than threats and bites." The Forest Troop

> . . . has maintained its genial style over two decades. [Apparently,] the resident baboons are instructing the immigrants in the unusual customs of the tribe . . . Hormone samples from the baboons showed far less evidence of stress in even the lowest ranking individuals when contrasted with baboons living in more rancorous societies. (p. 13)

What appears to have changed, according to the research, is a "social ethos of the group." It's an *attitude* that is being transmitted. One of the researchers suggested, "The good news for humans is that it looks like peaceful conditions, once established, can be maintained." The bad news is that "you might have to first knock out all the most aggressive males to get there."

On a more serious note, Martin Luther King (1987) once noted, "Every man (woman) must decide whether he will walk in the light of creative altruism or the darkness of destructive selfishness. Life's most persistent and urgent question is what are you doing for others" (p. 17). He also said, ". . . courage faces fear and thereby masters it. Cowardice represses fear and is thereby mastered by it" (p. 24). The RCT model might add that when we grasp the primary relatedness of our being, it may not have to be a dichotomous choice between altruism and selfishness. This opposition of self versus other is a construction of a competitive and dichotomous system, which cannot encompass complexity. By embracing a model of personhood that celebrates our interconnectedness, our need for each other, and our unending and inevitable vulnerability, we can see that the interests of other and oneself are far more intertwined than our prevailing psychological theories and social philosophies would lead us to believe. The practice of mutuality is at the heart of this convergence of interests.

I find hope in the process of healing the split that has been created between self and other, between self and society. I find hope in learning to live with complexity. I find hope in being *with* others in my vulnerability rather than standing *against* others in my "self-hood." I find hope in moving through the tension of fear to a sense of justice. As King noted, "True peace is not merely the absence of tension; it is the presence of justice" (p. 83) and "hatred and bitterness can never cure the disease of fear; only love can do that" (p. 90). Fear, without the possibility of moving toward others, is a place of darkness and isolation; hope created in connection brings light, clarity, and meaning. We are not alone, and we can make a difference for ourselves and for all people. Martin Luther King knew that, Gandhi knew that, Sojourner Truth knew that, Einstein knew that, Alice Paul knew that, and Rosa Parks knew that. Let us join in our commitment to remembering that truth: We are *not* alone and we *can* make a difference. Paul Friere (1999) wrote, "The pursuit of full humanity cannot be carried out in isolation or through individualism but only in fellowship and solidarity" (p. 72). Needing to connect is *not* a sign of weakness. In fact, connecting may be the most intelligent thing we can do in a culture of fear. Just as isolation is the glue that holds fear and oppression in place (Laing, 1998), connection fosters healing and courage, thereby releasing energy for social revolution.

REFERENCES

Altheide, D. (2002). *Creating fear: News and the construction of crisis*. New York: Aldine de Gruyter.
American Association of University Women (1993, June). *Hostile hallways*. New York: Foundation.
Angier, N. (2004, April 13). No time for bullies: Baboons retool their culture. *New York Times*, Science, p. 13.
Banks, A. (2001). Post-traumatic stress disorder: Relationships and brain chemistry. *Project Report No 8*. Wellesley, MA: Stone Center Working Paper Series.
Bowlby, J. (1973). *Attachment and loss, vol. 2: Separation*. New York: Basic Books.
Brown, L. (2003). *Girlfighting: Betrayal and rejection among girls*. New York: New York University Press.
Commission on Children at Risk. (2003). *Hardwired to connect: The new scientific case of authoritative communities*. New York: Institute for American Values.
Dalai Lama XIV, & Cutler, H. (1998). *The art of happiness: A handbook for living*. New York: Penguin Putnam.
Eisenberger, N., & Lieberman, M. (2003). *Why it hurts to be left out: The neurocognitive overlap between physical and social pain*. Unpublished manuscript, Department of Psychology, University of California, Los Angeles.
Foxman, P. (1996). *Dancing with fear: Overcoming anxiety in a world of stress and fear*. New York: Jason Aronson.
Friere, P. (1999). *Pedagogy of the oppressed*. New York: Continuum International Publishing Group.
Fuller, R. (2003). *Somebodies and nobodies: Overcoming the abuse of rank*. New York: New Society Publishers.
Gilligan, C. (1982). *In a different voice: Psychological theory women's development*. Cambridge, MA: Harvard University Press.
Greenberg, M., Carey, G., & Popper, F. (1985). External causes of death among young white Americans. *New England Journal of Medicine, 313*, 1482-1483.
Greenspan, M. (2003). *Healing through the dark emotions: The wisdom of grief, fear, and despair*. Boston: Shambahla. 9
Herman, J. (1992). *Trauma and recovery*. New York: Basic Books.
hooks, b. (1989). *Talking back: Thinking feminist, thinking black*. Boston, MA: South End Press.
hooks, b. (1994). *Teaching to transgress: Education as the practice of freedom*. New York: Routledge.
hooks, b. (2003). *Teaching community: A pedagogy of hope*. New York: Routledge.

Jordan, J. V. (1989). Relational development: Therapeutic implications of empathy and shame. *Work in Progress No. 39.* Wellesley, MA: Stone Center Working Paper Series.

Jordan, J. V. (1990). Courage in connection: Conflict, compassion, creativity. *Work in Progress No. 45.* Wellesley, MA: Stone Center Working Paper Series.

Jordan, J. V. (1992). Relational resilience. *Work in Progress No. 57.* Wellesley, MA: Stone Center Working Paper Series.

Jordan, J. V., Walker, M., & Hartling, L. (2004). *The complexity of connection.* New York: Guilford Press.

King, M. L. (1987). *The words of Martin Luther King, Jr.: Selected by Coretta Scott King.* New York: Newmarket Press.

Laing, K. (1998). Catalyst Leadership Workshop. *In Pursuit of Parity. Teachers as Liberators.* World Trade Center, Boston.

Luks, A. (1992). *The healing power of doing good: The health and spiritual benefits of doing good.* New York: Fawcett.

Merton, T. (1979). *Love and living.* New York: Farrar, Straus Giroux.

Miller, D. (1999). The norm of self interest. *American Psychologist, 54,* 1053-1060.

Miller, J. B., & Stiver, I. (1997). *The healing connection: How women form relationships in therapy and in life.* Boston: Beacon Press.

Mun Wah, L. (Producer/Director). (1994). *The Color of Fear* [Film]. (Available from Stir Fry Seminars & Consulting, 154 Santa Clara Ave, Oakland, CA 94610).

Norcross, J. (2002). *Psychotherapy relationships that work.* New York: Oxford University Press.

Panksept, J. (1998). *Affective neuroscience: The foundations of human and animal emotions.* New York: Oxford University Press.

Putnam, R. (2000). *Bowling alone: The collapse and revival of American community.* New York: Simon & Shuster.

Resnick, M., Bearman, P., Blum, R., Bauman, K., Harrris, K., Jones, J., Tabor, J., Beuhring, T., Sieving, R., Shew, M., Ireland, M., Bearinger, L., & Udry, J. (1997). Protecting adolescents from harm. *Journal of the American Medical Association, 278(10),* 823-832.

Schore, A. (2003). *Affect dysregulation and disorders of the self.* New York: W. W. Norton.

Shaw, D. (1994, September 11). Living scared: Why do the media make life seem so risky? *Los Angeles Times,* p. A1.

Stampp, K. (1989). *The peculiar institution: Slavery in the antebellum south.* New York: Vintage Books.

Taylor, S. (2002). *The tending instinct.* New York: Henry Holt.

Tronick, E., & Weinberg, K. M. (1997). Depressed mothers and infants: Failure to form dyadic states of consciousness. In L. Murray & P. Cooper (Eds.). *Postpartum depression in child development* (pp. 54-81). New York: Guilford.

Walker, M. (1999). Race, self, and society: Relational challenges in a culture of disconnection. *Work in Progress, No. 85.* Wellesley, MA: Stone Center Working Paper Series.

Walker, M. (2004, October). *Founding Concepts & Recent Development in Relational-Cultural Theory.* Paper presented at the Jean Baker Miller Fall Intensive Training Institute, Wellesley, MA.

Walker, M., & Rosen, W. (Eds.). (2004). *How connections heal.* New York: Guilford Press.

Van der Kolk, B. (1986). *Psychological trauma.* Washington, DC: American Psychiatric Association Press.

Von Garnier, K. (Director). (2004). *Iron Jawed Angels* [Film]. Warner Home Videos.

INDEX

Anxiety
    racism, and *see* Racism

Change 104-122
    "acting out" 114
    controlling images 104-122
    essence of life, as 105
    expertise, and 119-120
    impasses, and 115
    influence of patient 118
    initial session 117-118
    marginalized groups, and 121
    mutuality, and 104-122
    mutuality in movement, and 110-111
    power, and 104-122
    "power-over" forms of action 112-113
    RCT, and 105-106
    relational images, and 105-106
    relationship between patient and therapist 116-117
    societal context 106-108
    therapy, in 109-112
    threat of isolation, and 108-109
    threats to CIs 114
    "visionary pragmatist" 120-121
Changes in therapy 29-48
    central relational paradox 31
    change in essence of life 30
    "condemned isolation" 31
    controlling images 31
    influences 31
    psychological isolation, and 31
    relational images 30
    strategies of disconnection 31
    vignette one: Mary 32-38
    vignette two: Helen 39-43
    vignette three: Maura 43-48
Competence
    resilience, and 60

Connection
    resilience, and 61-62
Controlling images
    change, and 104-122
Creative moments 6-28
    central relational paradox 20
    characteristics 21-22
    co-creative moments 24
    condemned isolation 24-25
    creative change 23-24
    dangers to 26
    dominant-subordinate cultures, and 27
    growth-fostering connections 19-20
    importance of 26-27
    integrity of relationship 21
    interpretations, and 23-24
    meaning 7
    mutual empathy 20
    mutuality 25
    power-over conditions, and 20
    psychological isolation 20
    responsibility, and 22
    reversal of central relational paradox 25-26
    stages of therapy 22
    theory of therapy, and 19-21
    vignette one: Susan 7-10
    vignette two: Maura 10-15
    vignette three: Kirk 15-19
    welcoming of the new 24
Cultural disconnections 84-102
    assumptive frameworks of dominance, and 93-94
    authentic responsiveness, and 92-95
    authenticity, and 92-95
    binary framing of 91
    binary paradigm, fallacies of 90-92
    conflict and the "power-over" culture 87-88
    conflict as source of growth 89-90

cross-racial connection, and 99
everyday 95
exclusionary entrapment 91-92
growth, and 87
loss of relational accountability,
   and 91
multilayered power differentials, and 88
multiple social identities, and 87
mutuality, and 95-95
mutually empowering conflict,
   and 98
old controlling images of good
   therapies 97
"power-over" 87
power-over paradigm of therapy 88
racial socialization, and 93
reaction to 90
reactive paradigm of power-over,
   and 91
shifting vulnerabilities 89
therapy as work of faith 100
therapy relationship, and 86
unidimensional victim-hood,
   and 91
unwillingness to investigate 99-100
"victim-ness" 90

Existential anxiety
   racism, and 78
Expertise
   change, and 119-120

Fear 227-246
   "age of anxiety" 228
   altruism, and 243
   attitude 243
   commitment to connection, and
     227-246
   connection, and 234-236
   context to address 238
   creation of 229-230
   culture of 227-246
   denial of 230-233
   disconnection, and 234-236
   failures of mutuality 236
   manipulation of 227
   neurobiology of 234-236
   quality of presence, and 241
   RCT, and 236-239

relational-cultural model 233-234
relational possibility 238
self-interest, ethic of 231
"separate self" 232
social pairs 235
slavery, and 229
Sue's story 239-242
therapy 236-239
vulnerability, and 231
Feminist ethics
   power, and 148-149

Interpretation
   creative moments, and 23-24

Love
   vulnerability, and 222-224

Marginalization 182-201
   accommodation 185
   assimilation 185
   assessing risk in context of
     connection 189
   awareness 189
   connecting 189
   critical consciousness 189
   dynamics of power and
     privilege 183
   existing models of strength 186
   great lie of patriarchy 186
   matrix of domination 184
   naming 189
   new models of strength 190-191
   range of 183
   resistance 187-190
   shaming, and 188
   strength in vulnerability 191-192
   therapy 192-196
   transformative change 185
   vignettes 196-199
Mastery
   resilience, and 60
Miller, Jean Baker 3-4
Mutual empowerment
   resilience, and 58-59

Nonrelational world 158-181
   binary thinking 163
   continuum of connection 164

Index

cultures of disconnection 163
framework for building healthy
  resistance and resilience
  160-162
hierarchical cultures 165-169
  central relational paradox 166
  opportunities for change
    167-169
  traditional 165-166, 168
  vignette 1 166-167
normative socialization, and 159
opposition 176-178
  health options 176-178
  unhealthy 176-178
practices that promote or impede
  connection 165
pseudo-relational cultures 165,
  169-173
  illusion of connection 169
  opportunities for creating
    change 171-173
  vignette 2 170-171
RCT, and 158-181
reading working situations 162-164
relational approach to replacing
  non-relational practices 179-180
survival cultures 165, 173-176
  opportunities for creating
    change 175
  vignette 3 173-175

Power 123-138, 139-155
  "agreements" 150-151
  alternative model 136
  amplifying difference to expand
    relational space 134
  boundaries 148-149
  choosing relational accountability
    132-133
  cognition, and 131
  combining "opposites" 130-131
  complaint, and 135-136
  confusion in use of word 141
  creative moments in therapy
    146-148
  cultural legacy of 126
  default positions 153
  definition 123,124
  denial by white women therapists 144
  difference, and 126
  disavowal of 127-128
  disconnection, and 128-129,
    131-132
  dominant paradigm 127
  effectiveness, and 123-138
  engaging collaborative conflict 132
  envisioning alternate paradigm
    123-138
  exploring alternatives 150-153
  feminist ethics, and 148-149
  fluid expertise 146-147
  goals of therapy, and 145
  hidden 140-142
  hidden power in therapy 143-146
  historically marginalized
    people 126
  hoarding 129
  inequality, and 125-126
  mutual empowerment 133-134,
    145-146
  Native Americans, and 140
  negotiation 124-125
  obscuring realities of relationship 129
  patients' boundary violations
    152-153
  "power-over" 124
  practical steps in therapies 146-148
  practicing power of naming
    135-137
  practicing supported vulnerability 135
  presumed expertise 145
  preventing change 142-143
  RCT, and 123-138
  relational conflict 130
  resistance, and 141-142
  structural 141
  subordinates, and 143
  subverting power paradigm
    133-134
  telling truth about 139-155
  "The Principle Walk" 128
  underlying basis of boundaries
    149-150
  unilateral 126

Racism 69-83
  anxiety about racial difference
    70-71

existential anxiety, and 78
historical trauma of 71-72
Lauren's dilemma 72-75
natural anxiety, and 72
"one drop rule" 82
RCM, and 71-72
recognition of differences 71
relational healing 69-83
Sara's dilemma 76-82
slavery, and 72-73
toxic anxiety, and 75
tripartite model of anxiety 71
valuation based on skin colour 78-79, 80
Relational-cultural theory (RCT)
core ideas 2
creative moment *see* Creative moments
empathic failures 2
growth fostering relationships 2
power dynamics, and 3
recent developments 1-5
Resilience 49-68
ability to connect 54
African American mothers, and 54
assertiveness, and 55-56
children 55
competence, and 60
connecting intellectual and relational development 56
connection, and 61-62
cultural context 53
discrimination, and 58-59
flight or fight response 62
"good outcome", and 51-52
group esteem, and 57-58
"hardiness" 53-54
hardships, and 61-62
individual characteristics of 51
individual, relationally rethinking 54-55
intelligence, and 56
internal control, and 58-59
internal deficiency, and 59
internal locus of control (ILOC) 58-59
Jennifer and Julie case 63-65
Judith Jordan on 50
"life-giving empathic bridge" 50

mastery, and 60
mutual empowerment, and 58-59
parent-child relationship, and 55
popular construction of 51
quality of connection, and 63
RCT, and 52-53
relational experience, and 52
relationally tempered temperament 55-56
relational perspective 64-65
relational ways to strengthen 65-67
relationships, and 49-68
self-esteem, and 56-58
sense of worth, and 56-58
social esteem, and 57-58
social support, and 61-63
"special strengths" 52
strengthening 49-68
strengthening through relationships 63-65
stress resilience of white and black children 59
tend and befriend response to stress 62
"toughness", and 49
ways in which therapist may enhance 66-67
Resistance
marginalization, and 187-190

Self-esteem
resilience and 56-58
Shame
vulnerability, and 221-222
Social support
resilience, and 61-63

Threat of isolation
change, and 108-109

Vulnerability 202-226
acknowledging 210
boundaries 215-216
clinical vignette 216-221
courage in connection 204-206
disowned 207-208
dominant images of control 209-211
illusion of invulnerability 207-209

isolation, and 211-212
love, and 222-224
management of 219
meaning 206
mutual empathy 211-213
myths 209-210
new definitions of courage 202-226

political resistance, and 204-205
privilege of assumed safety 208
relational authenticity 214
shame, and 221-222
supported 207
therapeutic authenticity 213-214
valuing 202-226